*"...wonderful ...
probing/important...LCTC
the medical system... I highly recommend it."*

**—Morton Coleman, M.D.,
New York Presbyterian Hospital and the Cornell University Medical Center**

*"A great tool for consumers, brimming with practical tips for
how you can take charge of your health care."*

—Peter V. Lee, Executive Director, Center for Health Care Rights

*"A unique perspective that will aid health care consumers
who are forced to navigate complicated paperwork and
procedures in order to receive the health care they need."*

—U.S. Senator Patty Murray of Washington

*"The Lerners show patients how to assert themselves as
knowledgeable consumers—and receive courteous and
competent care. No one trapped in the thicket of today's
medical system should be without this guide."*

**—Peter Clarke and Susan H. Evans, Keck School of Medicine, University
of Southern California and authors of *Surviving Modern Medicine:
How to Get the Best from Doctors, Family, and Friends***

*"An excellent book—engaging, informative,
and very readable."*

—Robert Jenders, M.D., Columbia Presbyterian Medical Center

*"This brother-sister team has broken new ground in creating
a consumer-friendly book that's got it all. It's poignant,
provocative, practical, and participatory. . . . No one before
has created a 1-2-knockout punch with such clear and
easy-to-follow suggestions."*

**—David B. Nash, M.D., M.B.A., Jefferson Medical College,
from the Foreword**

Lerner's
Consumer Guide
to Health Care

Lerner's Consumer Guide to Health Care

HOW TO GET THE BEST HEALTH CARE FOR LESS

Paul Lerner

and Julie Lerner

L

LERNER COMMUNICATIONS, LTD.

"A Patient's Bill of Rights" reprinted with permission of the American Hospital Association, Copyright 1992.

Sample letters reprinted with permission of the Center for Health Care Rights, Copyright 1999. For more information, go to www.healthcarerights.org.

"Medical Checklist" and "Managing the Referral Process" reprinted with the permission of California Health Decisions, Inc.

Printed in the United States of America
Distributed by Independent Publishers Group, Chicago

Publisher's Cataloging-in-Publication
(Provided by Quality Books, Inc.)

Lerner, Paul (Paul Daniel)
    Lerner's consumer guide to health care : how to get the best health care for less / Paul Lerner and Julie Lerner ; foreword by David B. Nash. -- 1st ed.
    p. cm.
    Includes index.
    LCCN: 00-91157
    ISBN: 0-9669999-2- 4

    1. Medical care--United States. 2. Patient satisfaction. 3. Patients--Legal status, laws, etc.-- United States. 4. Consumer education--United States. I. Lerner, Julie. II. Title.

RA395.L47 2000   362.1'0973
                                      QBI00-528

10 9 8 7 6 5 4 3 2 1

DISCLAIMER

This book is designed to provide information about health care. It is sold with the understanding that the publisher and authors are not engaged in rendering medical or legal services. If medical services or other expert assistance is required, the services of a trained professional should be sought.

Every effort has been made to ensure that the factual material in this book is accurate. However, there may be errors, and information may have changed. In the health care field today, there are frequent changes in names, telephone numbers, fax numbers, addresses, and other data, and consumers will always need to check information for themselves. Inclusion of an organization or business in this book does not imply endorsement of any kind. The publisher and authors encourage you to gather as much information and advice as possible on your health care needs.

Lerner Communications, Ltd., and the authors shall have neither liability nor responsibility to any person or entity with respect to any loss or damage caused, or alleged to be caused, directly or indirectly by the information contained in this book.

Book design by Barbara M. Bachman

Contents

3. How to Get the Best Care from Doctors and Other Practitioners 77

Foreword

How can people get the best health care?

PAUL LERNER AND JULIE LERNER have ably addressed this question in *Lerner's Consumer Guide to Health Care*. After more than a decade of work in examining health care quality, I strongly believe that this brother-sister team has broken new ground in creating a consumer-friendly book that's *got it all*. It's poignant, provocative, practical, and participatory.

The book is poignant because it grows out of their personal and deeply held conviction that individual consumers can make a difference in improving the health care that they receive. Julie's struggle with cancer and Paul's efforts on behalf of patients with AIDS temper the entire tone of the book, lending it a conviction that is genuine and heartfelt.

It's provocative because, frankly, no one before has created a 1-2-knockout punch with such clear and easy-to-follow suggestions. The Lerners will soon learn that they have made many potential enemies on the part of hospitals, doctors, managed care organizations, and other insurance entities. No one likes to air dirty laundry in public, but the Lerners have done it in a caring and thoughtful manner.

It's practical because the book contains actual templates of conversations, phone calls, forms, and letters. There are even mnemonic devices and tips to help patients remember what kinds of questions to ask when they see their doctor or specialist. In a sense, this practicality enables the consumer to become his own ombudsman.

It's participatory because the Lerners have distilled the best work from national experts in such areas as learning how to protect one's self while a patient in the hospital. Using a note-book at the side of the bed as a kind of shadow medical record, the Lerners dissect the national disgrace of thousands of pre-ventable drug-related errors and dispassionately deal with the recent Institute of Medicine report about improving patient safety. All the information one needs to participate in a positive way in one's care is clearly laid out, even for the uninitiated.

The back of the book is packed with names, addresses, web sites, and telephone numbers to call for every conceivable disease, condition, and query from a consumer perspective. The book is a virtual "how-to" in terms of guaranteeing that one gets the best chance to receive the best possible care at the best possible price.

My hat is off to the Lerners in their attention to detail, and for the ring of truth in each of the clinical vignettes woven throughout the text. All of us, including health care profes-sionals, recognize that one day we will be patients. We are lucky that the Lerners have gone down this road before us and have provided a detailed and easy-to-read road map for the journey ahead.

DAVID B. NASH, M.D., M.B.A.
Jefferson Medical College
Philadelphia

Acknowledgments

We would like to thank Diane Aboulafia-D'Jaen, Kim Agle, American Hospital Association, Bob Arnot, M.D., Barbara M. Bachman, Stephanie Becker, M.D., Howard S. Berliner, Sc.D., Diana Bianco, Bookzone, Warren Brennan, Kelly Calden, California Health Decisions, Sharon Castlen, Center for Health Care Rights, Morton Coleman, M.D., Eleanor Dodson, Susan Dressler, CCAP, Murray S. Eckell, Charles Farber, M.D., Foundation for Accountability, Andrew P. Gessner, Harvey Ginsberg, Lisa Gomberg, Stephen Hartnett, Henry J. Kaiser Family Foundation, Howard Herzberg, Carol Hoenig, Independent Publishers Group, Rachel Ingber, Robert Jenders, M.D., Sherrie Kaplan, Ph.D., Deborah Kelly, David Klotz, Lesley Koeppel, Missy Krasner, John Kremer, David Lansky, Peter V. Lee, Dan and Lyn Lerner, Michael Lovelady, Ma's Bobbin Works, Scott Manning, David Marc, Curt Matthews, Jason Maynard, Scott Meyer, Suzanne Muntzing, Senator Patty Murray, David B. Nash, M.D., M.B.A., Jan Nathan, Sally Neher, Stephen Parahus, A.S.A., M.A.A.A., Bill Parkhurst, Ben Pesner, Publishers Marketing Association, Ann and Dirk Poole, Bobby Potterton, Dan Poynter, Robin Quinn, Gerard Raymond, Diane Robertson, Gregory Rodehau, Betty Rollin, Dana Gelb Safran, Sc.D., Dean Sandler, Jeanne Sather, Mark Scherzer, Will Schwalbe, Ellen Severoni, William Shernoff, Jeannie Smith, Marcella Smith, Mark Suchomel, Joe van Dyck, Mary Westheimer, and Ellen Yoshiuchi.

Thank you to all of the librarians, health and insurance department employees, consumer advocates, and health policy analysts around the country for your support, your willingness to share your expertise, and your efforts to help us track down information.

Many thanks go to the wonderful doctors, nurses, and other health practitioners and advocates we have met in the cancer and AIDS fields. Your skill and compassion have inspired us to help all Americans find the best possible health care for themselves and their loved ones.

For our grandmother,

Rose Lerner

Introduction

IF YOU ARE CONFUSED, frustrated, and intimidated by today's health care system—welcome to the club! It's a big club, and most of us belong.

The bad news is that the system is not likely to improve any time soon. The good news is that by being an informed consumer, you can get some of the best health care in the world. There are many steps you can take right now to save money, time, and frustration with medical services, insurance companies, doctors, and HMOs.

That's why we wrote this book. We want to give you real-life, easy-to-use information about getting the best health care by getting around the health care bureaucracy. This isn't theory, and it isn't politics. It's inside information that will help you now.

Like the characters in a novel by Charles Dickens, we live in the best of times and the worst of times when it comes to our health care. It is the best of times because of medical breakthroughs, technological innovations, and pharmaceutical discoveries that are saving lives and helping people live longer and better. It is the worst of times because our health care system is a mess—and getting messier all the time.

Trying to understand health care today is like driving a car without a dashboard. The engine sounds good, but you can't tell how fast you're going or whether you're about to run out of gas. We're going to give you a dashboard, so that you can navigate your way through the health care maze without crashing.

Why is this book necessary? Imagine going to a store to

get something you really need. Instead of helping you, the store employees tell you to sit down and fill out several long forms. Then they keep you waiting for an hour before they will let you speak. When you can finally tell them what you need, they say that you're wrong. They claim to know best. When you ask how much it will cost, they tell you they don't know; someone else will send you a bill in several weeks. Most of the cost will be paid by someone else, but you still may have to pay more than you can afford—and there's nothing you can do about it.

Would you go back to that store? Only if your life depended on it.

When the service is health care, our lives do depend on it. And so managed care companies, insurance firms, hospitals, and other medical facilities often treat us poorly, refuse to give us information, overcharge us, and become indignant when we ask simple questions.

It's time for a change. Our country has many very good doctors, but the system seems to be making it harder and harder to receive the best care. As a result, there's a growing unhappiness about health care in America. We frequently ask people what they think of the health care system. The most common answer by far is, "It's a mess!" In fact, when we did a survey of New York consumers last year, asking people to grade today's health care system in the U.S., respondents gave it an overall grade of C–. Only 4% gave it an A, 18% gave it a B, 34% gave it a C, and 22% gave it a D. Surprisingly, 14% flunked it altogether!

The sudden rise of HMOs and "managed care" has made the system unnecessarily complicated and frustrating. What is the difference between a POS and a PPO anyway? And why should you have to care about that if you get sick? And if we are living in an age of high technology, why do we get health care manuals that make no sense, receive bills that don't add up, and get stuck in voice mail hell when we call trying to figure things out?

There's no shortage of health and medical information in this age of data overload, 24-hour cable news, and Internet search engines. For an individual, though, it can be quite difficult to find pertinent information about health plans, hospitals, and other medical resources in your own community—and to make sure that you are getting the best care for yourself and your loved ones. So much of the material we get is irrelevant, obviously self-interested, or written in a jargon at least twice removed from normal English.

As things stand now, it's very hard to understand how health care works, much less where you can find objective and understandable information. Many consumers stop trying. It has become a cliché to say that most of us spend more time picking a refrigerator or a VCR than we do choosing a doctor, health plan, or hospital. This remains the case in spite of the fact that all of us consider our health to be more important than household appliances.

Problems with our health care system affect all of us. The United States is the richest and most developed nation in the world. However, we have a health care system that manages to be inefficient and expensive while still providing no health insurance coverage to 44 million Americans—including 11 million children. Politicians may talk a lot about health care, but the reality is that we consumers are the ping-pong ball in a game being played by HMO advertising executives, insurance industry PR people, and lobbyists and political operatives of all stripes. Although it's tempting to look for one Big Solution to this Big Problem, none is in sight on the political front. The best answer is closer to home. We all need to become patient advocates for ourselves and our loved ones.

You may hope that when you are sick, the health care system will be a cooperative place where your individual needs come first. But as a savvy consumer, you should know better. Increasingly, the inner workings of our health care system are like those of our legal system—adversarial, with different interest groups protecting their agendas. So you need to take responsibility for protecting your own interests.

Marcus Welby, M.D., is dead. In the Age of Managed Care, patients who "work the system" are more likely to get the best care. From our personal experiences, we've seen that being an assertive consumer—and even a "difficult patient"—is what works. Julie was a difficult patient, and that's one of the reasons she's still alive. We all need to stop being "good patients" and start being good consumers.

The two of us believe so strongly in this endeavor that we are willing to put our name on it—a rare thing in health care today. We are advocates for patients and health consumers only—we have no connections to insurance companies, HMOs, hospitals, or doctors' groups. Unlike most people in health care, we work solely for you, the consumer.

Some medical experts have told us that consumers are too intimidated, lazy, or dumb to use the information in this book to make good decisions about their health care. We think they're wrong. In the past decade, large numbers of Americans have taken control of their financial lives and begun investing for the future, greatly surprising the financial "experts." In the next decade, people will take control of their health care in similar ways. Learning from the patient advocacy movement, which has helped so many people affected by AIDS and cancer, we are on the verge of creating a new "individual health advocacy."

When enough of us have become informed and assertive consumers, the health care industry will have no choice but to respond to the changing marketplace. Our health care system will become more patient-focused—one consumer at a time.

Join us.

—Paul Lerner and Julie Lerner

1.

How to Get the Best Health Care

Julie Lerner's Story

IN THE EARLY 1990S, I WAS IN MY MID-TWENTIES, LIV-ing in New York City, and working at a radio station. I sold advertising for a commercial classical station that was owned by a large company. As an active young person, I enjoyed all of the good things of New York. I was happy, dating, and looking forward to marriage, kids—the usual goals.

I had been extremely healthy all my life. In 1990, before taking a trip to Europe (a belated college graduation present), I went to see my dermatologist because I had lumps on either side of my neck. The dermatologist seemed very concerned and said that I should have the lumps checked out.

So I went to a specialist. After taking an aspiration of the lumps, he said they were nothing. He remarked that they were probably due to hair coloring. That seemed odd, because I only highlighted my hair, never colored it. So for two years I went around with the false sense that the lumps in my neck were nothing to worry about. During that time, strange things started happening to me. For instance, I had chicken pox, and I started having immune system problems.

I later learned that this type of misdiagnosis is surprising-ly common. Many people are misdiagnosed when it comes to a serious illness. Medicine is a tricky thing, and it's more sub-jective than you realize. It's as much art as science.

It took a while for the pieces to come together. Eventually, they did. On May 5, 1992, I was diagnosed with a form of cancer called non-Hodgkin's lymphoma.

Two days later I saw a doctor to talk about treatment. I asked if I would still be able to have children. He responded, "Why are you worried about that? You might not live." Compassion and communication are not high priorities with all doctors, as I was to learn.

That was the beginning of my long journey into our medical system. From 1992 to 1996, I had nearly 30 inpatient stays and more than 300 outpatient visits at seven different hospitals around the country. In the process, I became a health care expert.

Though I hope you never need this information, I'm going to share what I learned about being a patient. At some point, you and your loved ones are going to face serious health issues. When it happens, remember this:

If you are sick, you've got to be tough, even when you don't feel tough. You've got to learn to rely on other people. It's almost impossible to go it alone, so look for support from family, friends, support groups, and not-for-profit organizations. You have to take the bull by the horns and find out information for yourself.

You should definitely get second opinions before you have a treatment. Let it be known if there are problems. Be vocal. Don't worry about being called "difficult." Take as much into your own hands as possible. Have friends or relatives by your side to act as your "patient advocate" during the times you don't feel up to it.

Write questions and comments down, in case you don't remember everything. Give these written questions and comments to your doctors and nurses, and make sure they give you answers. If you have problems in a hospital, contact the patient representatives—they will lobby for you.

Some doctors can be condescending. Don't let it get to you.

Don't be afraid to challenge your doctor. It's your life, and these are your decisions. If you search, you will find excellent doctors who are also wonderful, compassionate people. If you need to change doctors, do it. If you need to change hospitals, do that, too. It's your life—literally.

When your care involves a hospital stay, don't be surprised if the environment there is not nurturing. Hospitals can be cold and harsh. When I had cancer, I did not see myself as a "victim." But I often felt that I was treated like a victim in the hospital, and I started to feel like one. You may be facing the toughest moments of your life, but quite often the empathy is not there. Some of the doctors I dealt with were so cold that it was shocking to me. So I learned an important skill—how to change doctors.

Some medical experts may scoff when I talk about a "nurturing environment." After everything I've been through, I know that your environment can make a big difference in your attitude, and that your attitude can make a big difference in your health. You can make a hospital room more pleasant by bringing your own clothes, books, music, videos, pillows, and photographs. If the food is bad (and it often is), ask friends and family members to bring you food from somewhere else. Trust me, pizza will taste better than anything on the tray.

Going into the hospital may be an overwhelming experience, so do everything you can to make it easier on yourself. Now is the time to ask favors from friends, relatives, colleagues, and anyone else who can help.

After any treatment, there will be a lot of confusing paperwork. Keep good records. Start a file. Document everything. If you have a friend or relative who is good with numbers, enlist that person to help you keep track of your medical bills. The paperwork may go on for months. Prepare yourself—handling this paperwork can be a job in itself.

Which doctors and hospitals should you choose? Read and learn as much as you can. Talk to as many people as you can. Go visit hospitals to test what feels right.

I beat cancer with the help of good doctors, nurses, hospitals, friends, family, and good luck. Along the way, I consistently saw that it was difficult to find objective information about health care options, and I learned that you must be an assertive and informed consumer of health care. I realized that some institutions do not deserve their lofty reputations and that some people in the health care industry fail to put patients first. Most important, I learned that the real experts about health care are the patients—yet few people ask us our opinions.

I was particularly disenchanted with one hospital, which every year was rated #1 for cancer treatment by a national newsmagazine. At that hospital, I experienced condescending doctors, episodes of miscommunication, medical mistakes, bureaucracy, eight-hour waits for admission, and constant paperwork and billing foul-ups. Once a nurse yelled at me because friends were visiting my hospital room to cheer me up and we were all laughing. A person battling cancer should not be treated that way.

This hospital was a big bureaucratic machine. When you are facing a life-threatening illness, you want some element of humanity. While being treated there, I felt like a number. I was #988417. I will remember that number all my life.

I started to wonder who did all of these rankings regarding the quality of care. Were they ever patients themselves? No! In most surveys, they never even ask the patients. They talk to the "experts," not to the people who actually use the services.

When I was diagnosed with cancer, I was far from being an advocate. But after my experiences at this hospital, I became an activist. I went to the patient representative with ideas, but I didn't get anywhere. I asked to talk to the hospital's CEO, but could never get in. But I saw how things could be, and I started talking to other people who felt the same way.

I think it's time more attention was paid to the health consumer's point of view. That's one of the reasons my brother and I wrote this book. When I was diagnosed, I didn't have a lot of information to make good choices. I've learned that information is crucial, and I want every patient in the future to have more information so that they can make the best choices. Now, for me, it's about creating change.

I came very close to dying. I was given poor odds of surviving cancer—only about 15%—but I beat the odds. Recently I passed the five-year anniversary of my second bone marrow transplant. I'm officially in remission, and I'm doing very well. My long-term prognosis is excellent. I feel like I am one of the luckiest people around.

Today I'm a marketing executive in the restaurant industry. I love what I do. I'm active with the Cure For Lymphoma Foundation and the Leukemia and Lymphoma Society, and plan to walk a marathon soon for the Leukemia Society's "Team In Training." I also help people who are newly diagnosed with cancer and raise money for patient-aid programs.

I learned that every day of your life is a gift. After an experience like this, you really try hard to make it the best life you can. Now I don't wait to do things, whether it's walking a marathon, working for a cause, or writing a book.

People call me a survivor. I like that. I'm very proud of that word. My theme song is, "I Will Survive."

As a patient, I could only do so much. But now, I can do a lot more to help people. While facing my health challenges, I discovered how things work in health care—and how things often don't work for the patient. We as individuals have to be ready to stand up and demand our rights. The patients' point of view should be just as important as the "experts." That's why I've made it my mission to help other people find the best health care available—and not to let anything stop them.

Paul Lerner's Story

I lost friends to AIDS and then went to work in the AIDS field. In my five years working for not-for-profit AIDS service organizations, I found that the knowledgeable and motivated people with HIV were far more likely to survive and thrive.

I saw some amazing things while working with people with AIDS. As you can imagine, the work could be stressful and depressing because of the constant presence of illness and death. But it could also be surprisingly uplifting. While it's a difficult thing to see people facing death—especially when they are vibrant young people—it's also a very powerful experience to see individuals fight back, to reclaim their lives, to refuse to accept defeat, and to beat death. Sometimes they even did it with a smile.

One moment I'll never forget took place when I worked at an AIDS organization called Los Angeles Shanti, which provides support groups and other services for people affected by HIV. I had scheduled an interview with another staff member, David, for Shanti's newsletter. David had worked there for more than ten years, almost since the organization was founded. During those years, he had been diagnosed with AIDS himself, had gone through painful illnesses, had seen many friends and colleagues die, and had buried two lovers. At the time, I knew that David was suffering through neuropathy (nerve damage) in his legs, which made it painful to walk.

Despite all of this, he was one of the nicest, most pleasant, least bitter people I've ever known. I've met people whose biggest problem was a hangnail who complained about life more than David did. He seemed to take everything in stride.

During the interview, I asked him how he handled it all. How did he keep coming to work every day, helping people with AIDS, after all he had been through? He answered, "I think of myself as one of the luckiest people in the world, because despite all of the setbacks I've experienced, I've been able to help other people, and I've had so much love in my life. I'm in a new relationship now, and I feel very blessed."

I'll never forget that answer. It's a great approach to health and medicine. For that matter, it's a great approach to life.

I learned from David, and many others involved in the battle against AIDS, that being involved and aware can literally save your life. Averting your eyes from health problems and personal crises will not make them go away. On the contrary, confronting reality and educating yourself are keys to survival. As people often say, information is power.

What we saw with AIDS is that you have to be very assertive, and even aggressive, in taking control of your own care rather than expecting everything to work exactly as it "should." A big part of the reason we've made so much progress against the disease is that many people were forceful in doing patient advocacy and education. It's no accident that people with AIDS are living much longer now. And it's no accident that there are so many programs to help people affected by HIV and that the medical establishment takes AIDS very seriously now. None of those things were a given. At first, none of them happened. The federal government and many health authorities did not want to deal with this epidemic. We had to fight for each and every advance, step after step.

People with AIDS did a terrific job of informing themselves and forming community organizations. It really revolutionized the way people perceived health care. Doctors and patients shared information and listened to each other. People realized that they are entitled to a level of decent treatment. The response to AIDS became a model for all of health care.

It's time to take the sort of patient advocacy that has worked so well for people with AIDS and for women with breast cancer to the next step, which is the personal level. We call it Individual Health Advocacy.

That's what Julie and I do now. We encourage people to be patient advocates to make sure they get the best possible health care at all times. You can't take good care for granted. I'm afraid that you can't trust the health care system to do what's best for you. On a gut level, people know that. But quite often they are too afraid or intimidated to take positive steps to protect themselves. This book gives you the information, the tools, and the encouragement to take those steps.

Our health care system is dysfunctional, and it's not going to change any time soon. But we will help you "work the system" to get the best care, and to save money and frustration in the process. I learned a great deal during my years in AIDS advocacy; those lessons are shared in the pages ahead.

The Dirty Little Secret about Our Health Care System

Here's the dirty little secret about our health care system—we don't have one. Our health care is not in any real system. Rather, it's a patchwork of different programs, political compromises, government efforts, lobbying blitzes, ad campaigns, and outdated policies. It's many different systems that have built up over time, but which don't work together and don't communicate with each other.

It's a damn mess—but then, you knew that. This is what consumers have been telling us. Well, don't feel bad. The people in the system know that it's a mess, too. They just don't like to say it, because they fear that their words will be used against them in the power politics in Washington and the state capitals.

Astonishingly, the lobbyists for the health care industry like to claim that we have the best health care system in the world. Like many lobbyists, they keep their fingers crossed behind their backs as they speak. It's certainly true that we have some of the best doctors, hospitals, and medical researchers in the world. We are fortunate to have many brilliant and talented people working in American medicine. But a system is much more than the people who work within it. The truth is that we don't have the best health care system—on the contrary, we have one of the worst health care systems in the industrialized world.

You can't blame health care companies and politicians for

everything. We all need to take some responsibility, because we have continually said that we want more health care but don't want to pay for it. For instance, recent surveys by the Henry J. Kaiser Family Foundation found that 77% of Americans "strongly favor" making sure that all working families have insurance—but only 46% would pay more in taxes to get additional people covered.

We don't take policy positions, because our mission is solely focused on helping people get the best health care for themselves and their loved ones. If you want to get involved in the politics and policy debates of health care, we encourage you to do so. There are numerous organizations you can join and volunteer for; we list many of them in Appendix A. Whatever your views, make them heard. But make sure you understand where we are starting from. We hear too many people say, "If only the such-and-such program or law were put in place, then everything in health care would be great." That's not likely.

Much of the impetus for health care reform comes from people who would like to see us have a coherent health care system—whether a Clintonesque universal health insurance system, or a more free-market system where individuals make their own decisions with vouchers they receive from their employers or the government. Neither system is going to be instituted any time soon, because while everyone recognizes the current mess we are in, there is no political will to make fundamental changes. The attitude of the American public seems to be "the devil we know is better than the devil we don't know."

Most people are less interested in good health care policy than they are in making sure that good medical care will be available when it's needed by one of their family members. You want to know how to work this system (or perhaps we should say "work this mess"). That's what this book is about.

Once you realize that we don't have a health system, it shouldn't surprise you to find out that health care is not as tightly regulated as people think. We like to assume that some-one is carefully overseeing all medical care to ensure that every-thing works correctly. Like a lot of assumptions, that's wrong.

"Consumers have this idea that there is an organization that is maintaining a level of quality in health care," one expert told us. "They can't name the groups, but they 'know' it. It's just not so."

This lack of oversight and regulation extends beyond med-icine into the health care coverage you spend so much money on. According to Susan Dressler, CCAP, President of the Alliance of Claims Assistance Professionals, "For the most part, insurance companies are not regulated. State insurance commissioners have little sway over these people. There really isn't an organization that does that."

Being a consumer of health care is not nearly as much fun as being a consumer of televisions or stereo equipment, but it's a lot more important. Fortunately, there is great medical care out there. There are many excellent doctors, terrific hospitals, well-run health plans, and state-of-the-art medical clinics. Let's go find them.

Getting the Best Health Care

As we've discussed, it can be difficult to find even basic infor-mation about our health care options. Direct answers and good customer service are sorely lacking in the health care field. A 1998 Louis Harris poll for *USA Today* found that the three worst-rated industries for doing a "good job serving cus-tomers" were tobacco, managed health care, and health insur-ance. The health care industry was about as popular as a prod-uct that kills people!

Recent research has demonstrated that a positive attitude is very important for people facing serious health problems. How ironic, then, that the health care industry often treats people poorly and with a good deal of condescension.

After two years' worth of research into health care, we believe that some HMOs, insurance companies, and other medical businesses deliberately withhold relevant information and make material more confusing than it need be. They do not want us to understand everything they're doing, and they don't want us to be able to compare one company against another. For incomprehensible jargon, health care organizations take the lead. One health policy analyst told us about an experience in which he was baffled by his own insurance company's paperwork, adding, "And I'm an expert in this area!"

We don't buy it. Health care is a service industry, and it's time they provided better service. If enough of us demand that, they will be forced to improve. To learn how, read our section in Chapter Five titled, "Why Customer Service is So Bad—and How You Can Get Better Service."

We refer to all of the entities providing health coverage as "companies," even if they are not-for-profit. Whether or not the companies make profits, they still function as businesses. Health care is the largest industry in the country, with more than $1 trillion in spending every year. Yes, that is *trillion*.

Health care spending accounts for approximately 14% of the Gross Domestic Product (GDP) of the United States. That's bigger than the auto and software industries. As a health care consumer, you are a business customer—so demand good customer service. Some of us behave like the health care industry is still filled with selfless people who care only about our needs—when in reality we are dealing with harried employees of huge corporations whose CEOs make multi-million dollar salaries.

The health care industry counts on people being passive. One former HMO official says that she turned down many claims because she "knew as a medical director that very few people appealed claims."

It's not your fault that you can't understand most of what you are told by health care companies. Health care is complicated and confusing—on purpose. The health care companies want you to give up in frustration. We hear that phrase all the time. People tell us, "I gave up in frustration." *Don't.*

Become your own patient advocate. We know that you can do it. Recent surveys conducted by the not-for-profit organization Foundation for Accountability show that many people are eager to advocate for themselves in health care.

Being a patient advocate means that you will fight for yourself. You can't expect that the Customer Service Department at your health plan or hospital is there to help you. Quite often it seems that these departments are there to stop you from getting the services you need. Go in with the attitude that you know what is owed you, and that you're not going away until you get it.

Whatever you need in health care, fight until you receive it. If you are turned down for anything, appeal. If you are turned down again, appeal again. Make noise. Call your local elected officials. Call the media. Get as many people as you can on your side. Find allies. Recruit friends and family members to help.

Be ready to "go on strike against your health plan," to change your preferred hospital, or to fire your doctor. These are businesses, so treat them that way. We've got to stop letting the health care industry get away with this trick of being as profitable as a big business, as unaccountable as a private club, and as unhelpful as the worst government bureaucracy.

If only medical care worked as well in real life as it does on TV shows, where the doctors are always compassionate, the hospitals are always well-run, insurance coverage is always there for anyone who needs it, and medical mistakes virtually never happen and certainly never kill anyone. Then we would have nothing to worry about. But the reality is often quite different. (Memo to TV executives: We propose a program called *Patients,* about people who are forced to deal not only with illness but with an uncaring health system, yet who manage to survive and thrive.)

Health care should be more patient-centered. It is slowly moving in that direction, and the more of us who demand better service, the faster we will get there.

Demand the Best Care— You Have Already Paid for It!

You have already paid a lot of money for health care before you ever receive it. Think about all of the money you have paid over the years in monthly premiums, deductibles, co-payments, and taxes.

Yes, *taxes*—because a good portion of your taxes goes to pay for health care. Forty-two percent of medical costs in this country are paid by government agencies, funded by your tax dollars. All of that money goes for Medicare, Medicaid, Child Health Insurance Programs, military health care, the Federal Employee Health Benefit Program, and many other programs at the local, state, and federal levels. (By contrast, individuals pay 29.3% of total costs out of pocket, with the remaining 28.7% of health care costs paid for by companies on behalf of their employees.)

A recent census survey found that for the average middle-aged woman, health care is one of her largest annual expenditures. Health care spending now averages more than $4,000 per person every year.

This doesn't even count the tax breaks that companies get for providing health insurance to workers, a break that until recently has been unavailable to individuals. Companies get a big tax break, meaning that less money goes into the U.S. Treasury—so you're paying higher taxes to subsidize other people's medical care.

And not all of the money you spend for health care will go to protect your health. First there are the salaries. You may have heard of HMO executives who make millions of dollars a year. But did you know that many hospital administrators make six-figure incomes, with quite a few hospital CEOs earning more than half a million dollars a year? Or that among the more than 700,000 doctors in the United States, the average salary is nearly $200,000 a year? American doctors earn two to three times more than doctors in Western Europe. And despite doctors' complaints about managed care driving down salaries, *The Wall Street Journal* recently reported that doctors saw their salaries rise 47.4% during the 1990s.

Those are just salaries. Then there is marketing, promotion, advertising, and lobbying. Doctors spend more than $100 million a year on advertising. Insurance and managed care companies spend even more on marketing, as well as on lobbying campaigns against consumer-friendly legislation. In a good year, the managed care industry earns more than $20 billion in profit.

None of this counts the billions of health care dollars that are lost each year to waste, fraud, abuse, and outright theft. Even conservative estimates place this amount in the tens of billions of dollars annually, all of which ultimately comes out of our pockets in the form of higher charges. A recent report from the Inspector General of the Department of Health and Human Services stated that, in 1999, improper Medicare payments to doctors, hospitals, and other health care providers cost taxpayers $13.5 billion, approximately 8% of all payments in the traditional Fee-for-Service Medicare program. Another report from the same office found that taxpayers had paid Medicare HMOs millions of dollars for questionable expenses, including gifts, food, alcohol, and theater tickets.

So you can see that by the time you walk into a doctor's office, medical clinic, health center, or hospital, you've already paid a large amount into the health care system. Is this appreciated? No. What usually happens? They make you fill out lots of forms and scare you about how much money it will cost. Then if you get away with just a co-payment, you feel like you've gotten off the hook.

Quite a shell game, isn't it? You've already pumped thousands of dollars into the health care system during the last year, yet you're made to feel lucky to receive any services—much less good services.

Cost is a huge issue now. According to David Lansky, executive director of the Foundation for Accountability, two of the three most important issues for health consumers today relate to cost—medical costs and prescription drugs costs. (The third is getting access to preferred providers.)

Another way to think about it is this: Even if most of your health costs are subsidized by your employer, that's money that could be paid to you in wages if health costs weren't so high. This is your money on the table.

So the next time anyone in the health care industry gives you problems, remember that you're paying his salary. You're paying him well, and it's time for him to deliver.

And the next time you get a bill that's too high, get ready to negotiate. You don't have to accept every charge at face value. Almost everything in health care is negotiable, including doctors' fees, hospital bills, and insurance reimbursements. For more information, see Chapter Six, "How to Save Money and Find Free Services."

Know Your Rights

There's been a lot of talk lately about a Patient's Bill of Rights. We are for anything that gives consumers more voices and choices. But we also have to ask: What difference will a Patient's Bill of Rights make when most people know so little about the rights that they already have? Will this just be another document of which most people are unaware?

All Americans have rights in health care. Because there's relatively little oversight of medical care, it's up to you to learn what your rights are and to make sure you're getting what you deserve.

Most health care regulation has taken place at the state

level. Strong consumer protections have been legislated in many states, including Texas, New York, California, and Washington. Different states guarantee different things to health care consumers. For instance, did you know that New Yorkers in most health plans are guaranteed 15 paid visits every year to a chiropractor? Or that Texans can sue their health plans for damages? For details, contact your state health and insurance departments; we list information for departments in all 50 states in Appendix C.

Additionally, the professional associations and industry groups in health care, from the American Hospital Association to the American Medical Association and beyond, have their own internal codes of conduct that they expect members to follow.

When you stack it all up, you have a lot of rights in health care. But it's up to you to make sure that you receive what you should. Because of generally weak oversight and a lack of regulators, you will have to push the issue forward and get people on your side.

Some health care companies take advantage of patients by denying services and then confusing those who try to complain. Don't let them get away with it. If you have a problem with a doctor, health plan, or hospital, we suggest that you always try to deal with them directly first, but you can turn to a consumer group or government agency at any time. You don't have to wait until you are at the end of your rope. We've found that sometimes it's good to call an outside agency first, so that you know exactly what your rights are *before* complaining.

Sample Letter:
Complaint to a Government Agency

[date]

[address of government agency]

Re: [Grievance or appeal] against [name of health plan or medical group] OR URGENT APPEAL AGAINST [name of health plan or medical group]

[Your name], Subscriber #[your number]

To Whom It May Concern:

On [date] I filed an [appeal or grievance] with [name of health plan or medical group]. I am requesting the Department's assistance in resolving my difficulties with my [plan or group] because {select one of the following reasons why you are requesting the department's assistance}

I am not satisfied with the answer I have received from my plan to my [grievance OR appeal];

• My plan has failed to respond to my complaint, and it has been more than 60 days;

• IT IS AN URGENT SITUATION AND I NEED IMMEDIATE ASSISTANCE.

A copy of my [appeal or grievance] is enclosed. Please let me know if more information is needed. You may contact me at [telephone phone number].

Thank you, in advance, for your attention to this matter.

Sincerely,

[your name]

Enclosures: {Material and documentation you can consider attaching:}

Copy of [grievance or appeal], including attachments (medical records, letters from doctors, etc.).

Why Spending a Little Time on Health Now Will Save You a Lot in the Future

If you exercise and eat well, you will live longer and better. If you choose a good doctor and understand your health plan and local medical services, you will get better health care.

We know that the last thing that most healthy people want to think about is health care. But just like you plan ahead by investing for retirement and educating your children, here's an area where a little planning pays big dividends.

Dr. Sherrie Kaplan of the New England Medical Center advocates what she calls "Planned Patienthood." She notes that many people have taken the time to plan ahead for how they will get out of their home in case of fire—something that's statistically very unlikely to occur. Yet few of us take the necessary steps to make sure we'll receive the right medical care when we need it—even though every one of us will be a patient.

We research a health plan superficially when we purchase it, and then place the manual out of sight. Well, it's time to drag out that manual. Finding out what's covered by your health plan now could save you many frustrating phone calls and letters about billing and coverage disputes later. Let's be honest—it may take you a while to figure it out. As we've noted, health care companies write most of their manuals and contracts in "legalese" that's difficult for a layperson to understand. It often seems that the material is written by lawyers, then rewritten by insurance agents, and then rewritten again by doctors, until it's totally incomprehensible. But you will still learn a lot by reading the material and getting any questions answered ahead of time.

When we talk to people about their health care problems, one of the biggest issues we hear about is the failure to be reimbursed for medical services. Sometimes the health plan pulls a fast one, giving authorization for a service and then later refusing to pay for it because of "lack of medical necessity." But sometimes the situation is more benign; the consumer just assumed that the service was covered and went ahead without checking. Never assume. Contact your plan administration first and check. Saying "But I tried and the customer service line was busy" won't get your bill paid later on. Staying on the phone and checking ahead will save you all those phone calls you would make if you received a huge bill that you're not prepared to pay.

For complicated issues, you may need to make a few phone calls. Information gathering expert Matthew Lesko has a "Seven Phone Call Rule," meaning that it may take seven calls to get through to the right person. However, when you reach that person, you will get the information you need.

Health care companies don't make it easy for you. One expert we spoke to said, "Corporate denial is their strategy." They don't refuse services or coverage outright, but then again, they make the process so difficult that many people give up. All the more reason for you to beat the health care bureaucracy at its own game.

When you have a medical problem, preparation is even more important. We want to think that medicine is science and therefore everything is known and understood. But that's not the case. Much remains unknown about the human body.

If you have a serious illness or chronic condition, do as much research as you can on treatments. Even the best doctors understand that they cannot keep up with the flood of medical journals, studies, and articles that now appear. A good starting point is the web site of the National Guideline Clearinghouse at www.guideline.org. Listed are hundreds of guidelines prepared by medical specialty societies. The site is funded by the federal government, the American Association of Health Plans, and the American Medical Association.

"We recommend contacting good patient advocacy groups," says Diane Robertson, editor in chief of the Health Technology Assessment Group at not-for-profit health services research organization ECRI. "Always look for groups that have objective, unbiased information. Some advocacy groups have their own biases because of where they get their funding. There are many conflicts of interest in medicine—intellectual, financial, and otherwise."

Why Most People Don't Care about Medical Quality—and Why You Must

Most people don't care about medical quality.

Wait a second. Can that statement really be true?

Sort of. A more nuanced way to say it would be: Most people assume that they always receive the absolute best medical care at all times no matter where they go. Even though they know that some hairdressers are better than other hairdressers, and some accountants are better than other accountants, and some law firms are better than other law firms, they will refuse to even consider the possibility that there are differences in medical quality. So smart and sensible people, who would never hire an employee or a tax preparer or a preschool without extensive interviews and background checks, will nonetheless go and put their lives in the hands of anyone wearing a white coat.

Does that really make sense?

This sort of "denial" is understandable, because health care is quite intimidating and medicine is truly complex. The real problem, though, is the way that health care companies respond to this mass denial. They perceive that health consumers don't care about quality, so they don't have to focus on providing the best medical care.

Listen to Ellen Severoni, president of the not-for-profit group California Health Decisions: "Many a CEO of a health plan has said to me, 'Patients don't care about quality.'" She adds, "Patients don't talk about quality in the same way we do, but to think people don't care is a silly thing to say."

It's clear, though, that patients don't regularly express their desire for medical quality. And so health plans and hospitals often fail to emphasize medical quality—with potentially disastrous complications for you as a patient.

Here's an example: In several states, including Pennsylvania, New Jersey, and New York, the state Department of Health publishes very useful statistics about heart surgery. The statistics tell you which doctors and which hospitals have the best records for bypass surgery and angioplasty. The numbers also show who has the worst records, with the most patient deaths. The reports are free and easily available to anyone in booklet form and on the Internet. It's a gold mine of information. By using one of these reports, a heart patient could choose a doctor and hospital with an excellent record, gaining a significantly better chance of surviving a risky surgical procedure.

The report on Coronary Artery Bypass Graft (CABG) surgery in New York State in 1996, for example, shows the dramatic differences in survival. The hospital with the best record had a risk-adjusted mortality rate of 1.1%, while the hospital with the worst record had a mortality rate of 5.93%—meaning that patients were five times more likely to die at the second hospital. The report also shows why you want to go to a hospital that performs a "high volume" of the procedure or operation you're getting. The hospital with the most CABG surgeries had 1,814 cases and boasted a risk-adjusted mortality rate of 1.81%. A hospital tied for the least number of cases, at 94, had a mortality rate of 4.52%—more than double the death rate.

As valuable as these reports are, most heart patients never use them. Many are simply unaware of the information, but patients who learn about the reports often refuse to use them.

One prominent cardiologist told us that even many cardiologists do not pay attention to the reports, because they know that patients don't care.

We're not thrilled about reading statistics, and we know that most people feel the same way. Still, if they could save your health, it's worth looking at some numbers. Read the "report cards" about health plans and hospitals, and understand how they are compiled. Are they based on statistics for preventive care? On patient satisfaction? Or are they popularity contests where doctors rank other doctors and hospitals? Which is most important to you? What source do you want to hear from?

You might find that some doctors are dismissive about report cards and medical quality data. They don't like being ranked or evaluated—but then, who does? We didn't necessarily like getting grades in school or annual evaluations at work, but we learned from the experience. Medical quality is difficult to measure, but we're making progress. The health care industry will have to get used to report cards and rankings, because there will be a lot more of them in the future. That's good news for you as a consumer.

Some doctors and health administrators have resisted not just report cards, but systematic quality improvements in health care. Peter V. Lee, executive director of the Center for Health Care Rights, says, "Individual cowboy doctors have resisted innovations that occurred in other industries. There is not rigorous continuing training of all doctors, the way there is with airline pilots. It is truly phenomenal how many people get the wrong care."

The health care industry does not emphasize medical quality nearly enough. That's one of the reasons that up to 98,000 Americans are killed every year by medical mistakes in hospitals alone. (For more on this subject, read Chapter Four, "How to Get the Best Care in Hospitals.") One study of autopsies found that 40% of the deceased patients had died of advanced cancers that were never treated *or even diagnosed*. Doctors who treated these patients completely missed that the people had cancer.

Some courageous doctors and health care experts have been raising these quality issues for many years, risking their careers in the process. They have done great work in developing ways to define and measure medical quality. Still, their work has received far too little attention.

One area where consumers have made their voices heard is on denial of services, particularly by managed care organizations. This is an important issue, but it's only one issue. Being denied service is "under-care." Just as potentially harmful to you as a patient are "bad care," which is self-explanatory, and "over-care," where you are given too many tests and procedures. Over-treatment has risks for both your health and your pocketbook.

Ask questions about every test and procedure and find out why it is being performed. Sample questions include:

- Why is this being done?
- What are we looking for?
- Is there anything else that can be done?
- What will happen if this isn't done?
- Will this be painful? Is there any way to make it less painful?
- Are there any side effects? Is there any way to reduce potential side effects?
- Where can I learn more about this?

By reading this book, you are already on your way to being a savvy consumer of health care. Here's one area where you can be miles ahead of most people: Pay attention to medical quality, and demand the best for yourself and your loved ones.

Simply by understanding that medical quality varies and by actively taking steps to get the best quality, you will be more likely to receive the excellent care that you deserve.

Tell doctors, nurses, and health administrators, "I want to make sure that my family and I get the best quality health care." You will surely get their attention, because so few people ever raise the issue.

Saving money on health care is important, but medical quality is even more important. Peter V. Lee advises, "Look carefully at quality, not just cost. What is the cost of poor quality? The cost of being with a less-good surgeon can be quite high."

Recognize Good Health Care

This book is about how to get the best health care, and what to do when you have problems. We tell you to be tough and demand great care. Inevitably, we are focusing on difficult situations rather than on success stories.

So it's important to state that there is a lot of great medical care out there. When you receive good care, we encourage you to recognize it. Express your appreciation. Call just to say that you're happy with the services you received. Send thank you notes.

You may be surprised how seldom people working in health care get thank you notes or phone calls of appreciation. Doctors and nurses and other medical workers are human. They like to hear that they're doing a good job, and they will remember those people who take a few minutes to say thanks. They will be more likely to want to see those patients again and to develop a long-term professional relationship based on communication and trust. "Positive reinforcement is great for building relationships," one doctor told us.

Ultimately, recognizing good health care is just as important as fighting against bad care, and it's a lot easier.

2.

How to Get the Most from Your Health Plan

How to Choose a Health Plan (When You Have a Choice)

MANY OF US DON'T GET TO CHOOSE OUR HEALTH PLAN. OUR employer offers one plan, and that's it.

So if your employer (or association or union) offers you a choice, that's a good thing. At least it sounds good until you have to read those brochures and plan manuals, and actually must make a decision. A recent survey found that the average person spent 16 minutes looking over insurance materials before choosing a health plan. That probably involved trying to read some of the information before giving up, and then looking at the pictures of happy, smiling people talking to very attractive doctors. (Have you ever seen so many happy patients and attractive doctors?)

Don't believe everything you see. You know not to trust all of the Hollywood gossip and Internet stock tips you hear. Don't trust health care brochures and advertisements either. Read the fine print. One patient advocate told us, "Insurance companies are failing to educate people. They're afraid that if they tell people all of their rules, people might go to another plan."

Bring the same skepticism to health plans as you would to buying a car or major appliance. Think of it this way: Over the next several years, you will spend more on a health plan than on a major appliance, and perhaps nearly as much as you spend on a car.

If you have primary care physicians and specialists you want to keep, call their offices first. Speak to the billing manager to find out if they accept the health plan. Ask the doctor and office manager what they think of the plan. Find out what the financial relationship is between the plan and the doctor. Is capitation involved? ("Capitation" means that the doctor is paid a set amount per patient no matter what medical care gets delivered, giving doctors an incentive to deny care.) Does the plan pay its bills on time? Are they easy to work with?

If you are in a plan with "network benefits," you want to hear that your doctor is "in-network." If you are told that the doctors are "out-of-network" but that you can still see them for a higher fee, you need to understand that the cost could be much higher. A lot of people have been burned by UCR (Usual, Customary, and Reasonable rates), so find out as much as possible about how you will be reimbursed.

The same is true regarding any prescription drugs you're taking. Find out if a new health plan offers those exact drugs. Ask if the medication is on the "formulary" (list of approved drugs) and how much the co-payment runs. If your medications are not on the formulary, you may wind up paying most or all of the cost of the prescriptions—making that health plan a very expensive choice.

If you have a chronic condition, you'll want to ask even more questions. Find out how many specialists are available on each plan, what kind of educational support is provided, and whether rules on pre-existing conditions will affect you.

Ask your colleagues what they think about the different plans. (We list sample questions in the next section.) Talk to people who have had a lot of recent health care needs. If you ask someone who hasn't been to the doctor in two years, he'll probably say that he's very happy with his health plan—

because he's healthy! Ask people who are likely to have health care situations similar to yours. If you are a 30-year-old woman with three kids, then talking to a 60-year-old single man may not get you the information you need.

Talk to your employee benefits people. However, be aware that they may be reluctant to give you opinions. One journalist told us about an experience she had at her new job. The company's employee benefits person handed her several different health plan manuals, but absolutely refused to say anything about the options for fear of appearing "biased" toward one plan. We think that's a bit extreme. If the employee benefits person seems to be reluctant to give you an opinion, ask her what she's heard about other people's experiences. What problems have others had with Plan X? What did they like about it? How was the list of doctors and the customer service? (Don't ask for individual names or cases, because that would violate patient confidentiality.) Ask her what plan she chose for her own family!

It's worth getting benefits people on your side from the start. If you have a problem down the line with your health plan, you'll want to go back to them.

In addition to learning about other people's experiences, read report cards and look for unbiased information from independent sources. Your employer may give you outside material from sources including your state government and the NCQA (National Committee for Quality Assurance). If your employer doesn't give you this information, ask for it. You can also find material at your local library, on the Internet, through your local not-for-profit community health organizations, and by calling your state health and insurance departments. Ask your state insurance department how many complaints have been filed against the different health plans during the previous year. For information about managed care plans, you can contact the NCQA directly at (888) 275-7585 or go to www.ncqa.org.

Other independent sources of information are becoming more common. If you live in New York, you can use our consumer guidebook *Lerner Survey of Health Care in New York*. This book includes a survey of the major health plans and provides extensive information about hospitals and other medical services.

There are now web sites that give quality information about plans, such as www.healthgrades.com. If you are in Medicare, look at www.medicare.gov. Regional sites are also starting; for instance, Californians can look at www.healthscope.org.

What factors should you use to evaluate a health plan? According to the not-for-profit organization California Health Decisions, consumers use seven key values to judge their care: accountability, affordability, choice, dignity/respect, fairness, personal responsibility, and quality.

If you're considering joining a specific health plan, call it directly and ask it to send you unbiased rankings. If they won't send you information, that's a red flag that they may be trying to cover up their poor performance. Calling the plan will also give you a chance to check out its customer service—one of the greatest sources of customer dissatisfaction.

"When choosing a health plan, call the customer service lines and 'time' how long it takes for them to pick up the phone," says Diana Bianco of Consumers Union. "This is one good indication of how the plan treats enrollees." She adds, "The bottom line is that people have to educate themselves about how health plans work. If they have a choice, they should make an informed decision."

Is the plan for-profit or not-for-profit? The magazine *Consumer Reports* and the advocacy group Families USA have found that not-for-profit health plans tend to treat their patients better and get higher satisfaction ratings. This is especially true of not-for-profit plans which have been operating for many years and have built up a tradition of trust with their members. Additionally, not-for-profit health plans spend more of your premium dollar on actually providing medical care than do for-profit plans. At least one state, Minnesota, has banned for-profit HMOs.

We think that it's worth knowing whether health plans and hospitals are not-for-profit or for-profit. That being said, we encourage you to treat all health care organizations as businesses. Even not-for-profit companies can have a lot of profit flowing through them.

Finally, do try to read the plan manuals. We know, we know—they are boring and hard to read. Still, the manuals contain a lot of important information, and whatever material you absorb will give you an advantage when problems arise. At the very least, read the "Exclusions" section so that you know which services the plan won't pay for. You can also ask for a one-page "Summary Benefit" description giving the basics of each plan so that you can compare the choices.

When you have chosen a health plan, put its manual and marketing materials in a safe place with other important papers. You will probably need to refer to this information later.

Sample Questions to Ask Co-workers about Plans

- What health plan are you in now? Do you like it? How long have you been enrolled?
- Did you switch from a different plan? Why? What didn't you like about the old plan?
- Are there lots of good doctors on your plan? Was it easy to find one? Is it easy to switch doctors?
- Are there doctors' offices near where you live?
- What is the co-payment for an office visit?
- Are preventive and "well visits" covered?
- Have you had any billing problems with the plan?

- What is the co-payment for a prescription? Is it easy to get filled? What pharmacy do you use? Can you get prescriptions by mail order?
- Is it easy to get referrals? How long do you have to wait?
- Are there enough specialists in the plan? Are the specialists top-notch?
- Are there enough doctors in the network? Have you gone out of the network? How much did that cost?
- How is customer service? Can you get questions answered? Do they respond to problems?
- Has the plan changed the cost of its co-payments recently? Do doctors drop off the plan a lot?
- Do you know what hospitals the plan is affiliated with?

If Only One Plan Is Offered, Get the Most Out of It!

If you are only offered one health plan, you are in the same situation as millions of other Americans.

Fortunately, there is one important choice you still have: which doctor to pick. You may just be handed a list of names and told to choose one by a certain date. Don't pick blindly. If you can't change health plans, your relationship with your doctor is vitally important.

You want to have a doctor who communicates well with you, responds to your needs, and is available when you need care. For tips on picking a doctor, see "How to Choose a Doctor from a List," the first section of Chapter Three.

If you have a doctor who is not helpful and responsive, change doctors. Most health plans make this fairly easy to do. Do it now—before there is an emergency or a serious condition.

Find out what your health plan offers in terms of free and low-cost prevention programs, and take advantage of as many as you can. Does your plan or company offer any discounts for fitness centers, wellness workshops, and nutritionists? Use them.

If an employer-provided health plan is not meeting your needs, then it's time to talk to your friends in the employee benefits department. If co-workers have told you they don't like the plan either, that's all the better. Try to bring these co-workers into a meeting, or at least write down their comments. Bringing co-workers into the discussion will lend support and reduce any fears you might have about discussing your concerns. Tell the employee benefits people, "This health plan is not working for me, and other people have told me it's not working for them. Can we find a way to improve it? If not, can the company switch to a new plan next year? When could that happen? This is really an important thing for a lot of us working here."

Employers are sensitive to this type of complaint, because the company spends a lot of money on the health plan—and because it wants its employees to be healthy and productive. Health care is usually the most expensive and most important benefit provided to employees. In a tight labor market, it's an important factor in hiring and retaining good employees. If your company calls the health plan to complain, that carries a lot more weight than if you call as an individual.

How to Find an
Individual Health Plan

Our society prizes individuality—except in health coverage. Dealing with health plans is not easy for anyone, but it's particularly difficult for an individual seeking coverage.

If you have looked for an individual plan—because you're a freelancer, independent contractor, employed but lacking coverage at work, or for any other reason—you know how hard it can be. Sometimes you simply can't find coverage. For example, as of this writing, not a single insurance company directly offers individual health coverage in the entire state of Washington.

Even if you can find individual coverage, you will probably pay much more than your friends in group health plans. So your best approach is to get on a group plan, which may be easier than you expect. Look into all the groups you can join, including associations, alumni organizations, churches, and professional groups. Many of these groups already offer a health plan at a reasonable rate. The plan is likely to be a managed care plan rather than a Fee-for-Service plan, but then most people who are covered through work no longer have access to Fee-for-Service, either.

Working Today is the name of an association for the self-employed that offers a health plan in the New York City area and may expand to other regions. It can be reached at (212) 366-6066 or www.workingtoday.org. People in the arts community can learn about low-cost coverage through the Artists' Health Insurance Resource Center at (800) 798-8447, and anyone can use the Center's informative web site at www.actorsfund.org/ahirc.

For an informative and helpful explanation of your rights to purchase individual health care coverage in each state, look at the web site of Georgetown University's Institute for Health Care Research and Policy at www.georgetown.edu/research/ihcrp/hipaa.

You can contact insurance agents, although many will not deal with the individual health insurance market. If they do, their recommendations may be influenced by their existing relationships with insurance companies and by the type of commission they receive for selling policies. If you already have homeowner's, auto, or some other type of insurance, contact your insurance agent for information or referrals. You can also find an independent agent (who works with many insurance companies) through the Independent Insurance Agents of America at (800) 221-7917 or www.independentagent.com.

You may want to look into large insurance companies that provide health coverage nationally, if only to check on their prices. For instance, you can check on prices and availability of PPOs from Mutual of Omaha at (800) 775-6000 or Fortis at (800) 211-1193. You can also inquire about an MSA (Medical Saving Account), a policy offered by some insurance companies that combines a medical insurance plan with an investment account.

Also check out government regulations. A good first step is to call your state health department. In some states, health plans must accept anyone who applies for coverage ("open enrollment") at set premiums ("community rating").

If you have a major pre-existing condition, 29 states offer "Risk Pools" so that people with cancer, AIDS, and other serious conditions can get coverage. The not-for-profit group Communicating for Agriculture has a list of risk pools on its web site at www.cainc.org. The group also publishes a national reference book titled *Comprehensive Health Insurance for High-Risk Individuals*; check your library or contact the group at (800) 432-3276. (Many farmers are self-employed and have found it difficult to find health coverage, thus the name of the organization.)

Get health insurance coverage of some kind. Far too many people go without it. Currently, 16% of the population has no health insurance coverage—and the numbers are climbing steadily. Some low-income working people feel that they just cannot afford health insurance. We recently spoke to a chiropractor in Washington, DC, who told us that even she did not have health insurance because she could not currently pay for it.

Surprisingly, though, 8 million uninsured people live in households with an annual income of more than $50,000. They are making a lifestyle choice that they would rather spend their money on other things instead of health insurance.

As the old saying goes, you could get hit by a bus any day. Or let Julie give you a word of caution: "Don't think that just because you're a young person, you don't need health insurance. I was 26 and had just gotten a job with a big company that had excellent health coverage. Then I was diagnosed with cancer. If I didn't have that good insurance, I might be dead now. I've seen many young people who didn't have health insurance, and you can get into very scary situations."

Or let your family members tell you why you need health insurance. When we published our guidebook to New York health care, we noticed that we got a lot of orders from outside New York. When we asked these people why they were buying the book, the answer was usually something like, "My son lives in New York and he doesn't have any health coverage, and I have to find him a health plan."

If you have small children, then at the very least obtain health coverage for them. Call the Child Health Insurance Program (CHIP) Hotline at (877) KIDS-NOW to ask about subsidized plans for children up to age 18.

When looking for individual health coverage, a good tactic is talking to other people with similar career and family situations. For instance, if you're a freelance graphic designer, talk to other designers. Learn about local and national associations of freelance graphic designers, and call their offices. (The Graphic Artists Guild offers a health plan.) Check out newsletters and web sites targeted to graphic designers. And if you need to broaden your search, ask freelancers in other fields where they found health coverage.

Sample questions are listed below.

Sample Questions to Ask Friends and Colleagues

- I need to get on an individual health plan. What do you use?

- Do you know anyone who has health coverage that's not from his workplace?
- Do you know of any health plans that accept individuals? Any that are affordable?
- Are there any community health organizations around here that I could call to ask about health coverage?
- Are there any trade associations that offer group plans? What are the plans like?
- Beside the plan that you joined, were there any others that sounded good? Why did you join that one? How has it worked for you?
- Do you know anyone else I could ask about health plans?

Know Your Health Plan

Many people don't know what type of health plan they're in.

People approach us regularly to discuss problems with their plans. Our first question is to ask what type of plan they have. Commonly they respond by giving the name of the company that provides the plan, like "Blue Cross" or "Cigna." (There are hundreds of companies providing health care plans in the U.S., but the largest are Aetna U.S. Healthcare, United HealthCare, Cigna, Foundation Health Systems, PacifiCare, Wellpoint Health Networks, Kaiser Permanente, Oxford, Humana, and the Blue Cross and Blue Shield companies within each state.) We have also talked to people who insisted that they were not in an HMO and then described their health plan—which was clearly an HMO. Apparently the bad press for HMOs has made people not want to even *think* about being in one.

To get the best care, understand what type of health plan you have. There are four major types:

1. HMO (Health Maintenance Organization). This is a type of managed care where you are limited in your choice of doctors and hospitals. In return, HMOs often pay more of the charges (requiring only a $10 co-payment, for instance), don't use claims forms, and say they emphasize preventive care. There are different kinds of HMOs (different "models" of care). The most common are the Staff Model (in which doctors are employees with a fixed salary), the Independent Practice Association Model (or IPA, in which doctors contract with several HMOs, usually for a set monthly fee per patient), the Group Model (which falls in between the other two), and the Mixed Model (which mixes the previous three). Some observers advise people to find a Staff Model, because theoretically a doctor in this system has no incentive to deny care, where a doctor receiving a set payment may "undertreat" patients in order to make more money. But other experts report that if you want to develop a long-term relationship with an HMO doctor, an IPA Model is better. Most HMOs are primarily business arrangements, not ways of providing care or overseeing doctors.

HMOs have gotten a lot of negative publicity lately, but many people have found them a convenient and cost-effective way of receiving medical care. The five biggest complaints about HMOs, according to the Center for Patient Advocacy, are access to specialists, arbitrary managed-care policies, access to and coverage for emergency room care, getting information about plans, and bureaucracy. A 1994 study found that HMOs provided better coordination of care at a lower cost than Fee-for-Service plans, but that HMO members received less comprehensive care and had a weaker doctor-patient bond.

2. POS (Point of Service). This comes as an option from managed-care companies. If you stay within the network, your charges are paid to the same extent as in the HMO. But you can choose to go "out-of-network," that is, outside the system, to other doctors or hospitals—if you are willing to pay more for the visit. The cost to you could be significantly more, because your plan will only reimburse providers according to its "Usual, Customary, and Reasonable" (UCR) rate, and there will be deductibles. Your monthly premium for a Point of Service option is usually higher as well. Ask yourself how much flexibility you want, and how much you are willing to pay for it.

3. PPO (Preferred Provider Organization). This is a modified type of Fee-for-Service plan. You go to a doctor in a network, who is a "preferred provider," and pay either a co-payment or a small percentage of the bill. If you go to a doctor outside the provider network, you pay more (perhaps much more). A PPO is sometimes referred to as "managed Fee-for-Service." It is similar to Point of Service, but often provides more flexibility than a POS plan.

4. Fee-for-Service. This is the type of health insurance many of us had before the rise of managed care. In Fee-for-Service, you make the decisions. You can go to any doctor, specialist, or hospital you want. After you have reached the limit of your deductible, the insurance company pays most of the bill, and you pay the rest. (For instance, after you spend $250 out of your pocket to reach the deductible, the insurance pays 80% of costs, and you pay the other 20%.) It is truly an insurance plan, as opposed to an HMO, which is a "prepaid" health plan. The advantage is obvious: maximum choice. The disadvantages: lots of paperwork, your 20% can add up to a lot of money, and the plans are becoming much harder to find and keep.

Why is it hard to find Fee-for-Service plans, and why are they so expensive? These plans became rife with abuse and "over-care." Because doctors, medical clinics, and hospitals were reimbursed for each visit or test, there was a fleecing of the system. Some providers really soaked the insurance companies, and even honest practitioners became used to ordering numerous tests "just in case." Yet even with all that expense, Fee-for-Service plans did not provide effective medical management of patients. "Managed care" emerged not just to cut costs, but to provide greater coordination of patient care. In 1984, 95% of people receiving health coverage at work were in Fee-for-Service plans. By 1999, only 17% were.

Need to choose a health plan? First find out which types are available to you. Then decide how much flexibility you want in choosing providers (doctors and other practitioners). HMOs are the least flexible (and often the least expensive), while Fee-for-Service plans are the most flexible (and often the most expensive).

FLEXIBILITY OF HEALTH PLANS

Least Flexible . . . . *Most Flexible*

HMO   POS   PPO   Fee-For-Service

Least Expensive . . . . *Most Expensive*

If you are confused by this alphabet soup of information, don't worry—most other people are as well. In the early 1990s, most of us hadn't even heard the term "managed care," even though HMOs had existed for decades. Now the vast majority of us are in some form of managed health care. This rapid shift occurred for many reasons, but chances are that no one told you what was going on. Diana Bianco of Consumers Union notes, "When managed care started to take over, a perfectly horrific job was done in informing people about their health care. One day people woke up, and the way they got their health care was different."

We all know that there has been a backlash against HMOs.

Still, we're not going to go back to a system where most people had Fee-for-Service insurance because those plans are very expensive. So let's adjust to managed care and make it work for us rather than against us.

One patient advocate told us, "HMOs are for people who understand what they're getting. These plans work well for people who follow the rules. But if you don't understand the rules, then you are going to be denied services." William Shernoff, a Claremont, California-based lawyer who has represented many health consumers, says, "If a consumer is really educated and knows how HMOs work, he can do a fair job of maximizing the chances of getting the treatment he needs. That starts with investigating the HMOs at the start and choosing one with a large panel of specialists. The more specialists they have, the better."

If you are in a managed care plan, ask your doctor how he gets paid. Why should you care? Because it can affect the amount of care you receive. In some states, including California, Colorado, and Texas, many managed care plans are putting all treatment decisions in the hands of the doctors. That sounds good, right? The problem is that plans are also giving the medical practices a set amount of money per patient per month. This is capitation, and it means that the medical practice takes the "risk" of a patient having serious medical issues that cost them far more money than they're receiving to care for that patient. To understand what this can mean, consider that a medical practice recently went bankrupt when one of its patients required several complicated surgeries.

As we mentioned, some experts believe that capitation gives doctors an incentive to deny patients care. After all, they point out, if doctors provide a lot of care, the money is coming right out of their pockets. Consumer advocates call these kinds of medical practices "HMO-itos," and question the ethics of doctors getting paid this way. Shernoff says, "It's a terrible system. The bottom line with capitation is that the less medical care they give, the more profit they're going to make. They give incentives to doctors and administrators to deny care; that's why they have all these treatment reviews set up." We have heard reports that some doctors refuse to accept capitated plans because of the risk of losing money.

Another tactic is to reward doctors who spend little money on their patients. If a doctor keeps spending below set limits for things like referrals to specialists and hospitalizations, the doctor receives a bonus. The bonus amounts can range from hundreds to many thousands of dollars. "Medical kickbacks" is what some consumer advocates call it.

You can ask your doctors how they get paid. Doctors may not be comfortable discussing financial issues, but questions about cost are perfectly appropriate, particularly in this day and age. After all, it's your money, and it's your life.

A Note About Self-Funded Plans: We have encouraged people to understand the health care rights they have in their state, and to call on local resources whenever needed. There's a big exception, though: self-funded plans. Many large employers fund their own health insurance plans, taking the "risk" on themselves. They still offer the types of plans listed above (HMO, PPO, etc.), but because of a complicated federal law called ERISA, the plans are not subject to state regulation. Instead, they are regulated by the federal government—and loosely regulated at that.

Approximately 48 million people are enrolled in self-funded plans. The bad news for these people is that those new state laws don't currently help them. If they have a problem in a self-funded plan, they cannot turn to state regulators, and it's harder to win an appeal at the federal level.

The good news for people in self-funded plans is that ERISA, which stands for the Employee Retirement Income Security Act, has its own consumer protections. Under ERISA, it's the obligation of health plan administrators to act prudently. They have a fiduciary duty to operate the plan in the interests of beneficiaries. They must provide a considerable amount of information about the plan and claims processes, and must give a "full and fair review" if benefits are denied. The plan has time limits on deciding claims and must give written explanations of its decisions in a manner that you can understand.

For more information about ERISA, contact the Pension and Welfare Benefit Administration (PWBA) of the U.S. Department of Labor. A list of national and regional PWBA offices is in Appendix D. If you are in a self-funded plan and have a problem, try contacting someone in a regional office first.

After all those details and initials, here's some good news: The rise of managed care has brought much more discussion of the importance of prevention programs. Some plans have implemented the programs, while others have done more talking than preventing. But overall it has become easier to get access to paid physicals, cancer prevention examinations, smoking cessation, weight management, and healthy living workshops.

Take advantage of prevention programs and other free services offered by your plan. If you don't, you are leaving money on the table. You have paid for those programs with your health insurance premiums. If you get coverage through work, your employer has paid as well—with money that could have been given directly to you but is instead used to subsidize a valuable benefit for your health. By passing on these offerings, you are also increasing the cost of your future health care, because health conditions that are prevented or caught early are much more easily and affordably treated than those found late.

Here's a simple five-step device to remind yourself about these services, using the acronym CURES:

Choose to be a key part of your own "health care team."
Use all of the preventive care programs you can.
Receive every physical you are entitled to have.
Educate yourself about what's in your health plan.
Search out the best doctors and services for your needs.

On that last point, searching out the best doctors, the good news is that you can find excellent doctors in managed care plans. Years ago, some good doctors refused to join managed care networks. Patients heard that you couldn't get the best doctors in managed care plans and that HMOs were filled with "second-rate" doctors. We don't know if that was ever really true, but it's certainly not the case now. Managed care has become so pervasive that very few doctors can avoid being part of some networks. More than 80% of primary care physicians have at least one managed-care contract, and most of the best doctors are in managed care.

Having a good relationship with your doctor is a very important part of your health care. But being in a good health plan, and knowing how that plan works, is nearly as important. Most patients have the notion that their doctor makes all the decisions and is responsible for all of their care, while the health plan merely pays the bills. David Lansky of the Foundation for Accountability refers to this notion as the "permafrost" in the health consumer's consciousness, because it is so difficult to break through.

He adds, "No one doctor can master it all. Your doctor needs help and support from colleagues, technicians, and managers to bring the right knowledge to you. Managed care and medical groups sometimes do that—that's the hope. Don't get fixated on the idea that your doctor should be a solo cowboy with no oversight or support."

Knowing how to work your health plan ultimately means that you are more likely to get the best care. A consumer expert told us, "People have to educate themselves about what coverage they have. If you buy an appliance, you have to learn how to use the equipment. Part of that is following the rules that are set out. A lot of people don't even know what kind of insurance they have. They haven't read, or haven't been given, their plan policy. The big thing now is education."

Another factor you may want to examine is your plan's financial health. Because a few health insurance companies have gone bankrupt or suffered serious financial problems, some consumers feel worried about their plan's long-term prognosis. If you want to check on a company's bottom line, you can easily get information from the leading ratings firms, including:

- A. M. Best, www.ambest.com
- Duff & Phelps, www.dcrco.com
- Insure.com, www.insure.com/ratings (an Internet service that lists ratings from other firms)
- Moody's, www.moodys.com
- Standard & Poor's, www.standardandpoors.com/ratings/insurance
- Weiss Ratings, www.weissratings.com. Or call (800) 289-9222; you will be charged a fee for a report mailed to you.

Ratings information is also available at libraries and through your local insurance agents.

Finally, there is a way to really improve your health plan. If you are committed to improving the care and service, get directly involved in the plan's operation. Many plans have consumer committees; some states require them to do so. This type of consumer participation makes a big difference.

According to Ellen Severoni of California Health Decisions, one of the biggest problems with health plan administrators has been that "they talk to themselves too much. More consumers could begin to ask their health plans, how are you involving other consumers? Some companies have very involved and engaged advisory committees, which work to make changes. One of the reasons managed care suffered such a backlash is that nobody invited me, the consumer, to the table to talk about it. All of those decisions were made behind closed doors. Now it's time to engage consumers."

How to Get a Referral to a Specialist

GETTING REFERRALS TO specialists is one of the most serious problems faced by health consumers today. We hear all the time from people who feel frustrated that they cannot get the referral they need, or go to the specialist they want, or make an appointment in a reasonable amount of time. The problem is especially acute for potentially expensive treatments in areas such as mental health, allergies, and rare conditions.

Dealing with a "gatekeeper" causes the most complaints. The gatekeeper is usually your regular doctor, known as your primary care physician. Managed care plans say that gatekeepers provide more coordinated care, so that the patient receives more focused and effective treatment. There's some evidence to support this contention. But many people suspect that the real intention of gatekeepers is to keep patients away from expensive specialists. Fortunately the most restrictive kinds of managed care plans are becoming less common, and more plans are allowing patients direct access to specialists.

If you really need a specialist, don't let anyone stand in your way. You have a "medical necessity." This is the term managed care companies use to approve (and sometimes deny) care, so you should use the term as well. If a treatment is a medical necessity, your health plan has a contractual obligation to pay for it.

A common problem is getting a referral to a specialist shortly after you've changed health plans, before you've had a visit with your primary care physician. One tactic to minimize this problem is to schedule a physical or well-visit with your primary care physician as soon as you join the new plan. During the visit, discuss your existing relationship with the specialist. That way the plan has a chart on you, and the chart mentions your condition and the specialist.

You can also call the office manager in your specialist's office to let her know that you've changed plans and may need help in continuing the relationship. The office manager may be able to intercede on your behalf.

Most things in health care are negotiable, including the service coverage from health plans. For instance, if your coverage for a particular kind of treatment has run out (say that you were entitled to 10 visits to a chiropractor and you've used them all up), ask your health plan about "flexing your benefit." That means giving up a benefit you're entitled to (mental health treatment, for example) but probably aren't going to use so that you can get more of a benefit that you really need (like additional chiropractor visits).

We have heard people complain bitterly about having to wait to see a specialist. If this happens to you, ask yourself, how severe is my condition? How quickly do I really need to see a specialist? Most of us don't like to wait. However, if your condition is not urgent, then waiting a few weeks probably won't matter. You would prefer to see the doctor earlier, but it's not an overwhelming burden.

On the other hand, if your condition is urgent, you're in severe pain, or waiting for treatment could cause a condition to seriously worsen—then you should demand priority scheduling to see a specialist. Use words like the ones we just did. Say "I need priority scheduling to see a specialist for urgent care, because this is a medical necessity and if I don't get treatment my condition could seriously worsen." That will work far better than simply saying, "I don't feel well."

You can also raise the bar by saying, "It's better that I see a specialist tomorrow than wind up in the emergency room in a few days." One doctor told us flatly, "Use the word *emergency.* It will get a different response."

Try to be nice, but always be persistent. If you are dealing with a doctor's receptionist, remember that she's often doing eight things at once. If you can't get any satisfaction, ask to speak to the office manager. Ask if they have contacts at the health plan or wherever the hold up is coming from.

If you don't feel well enough to push the issue, get a relative or friend to do it for you. Write down everything that happens. Use the following checklist to "manage" the referral process. Quite often, appointments are slowed down because of simple paperwork snafus on the part of the doctor or the patient.

After all that, if your health plan or medical group is not being responsive, send a brief letter stating the situation and asking for immediate care. You can use the sample letter later in this chapter as a starting point. Fax the letter, send it by express mail, or send it by certified mail with a return receipt.

Make sure to send copies of the letter to government agencies, and put their names at the bottom of the letter following "cc:" to indicate that a copy has been sent. That will get the attention of your health plan or medical clinic. It's true that the squeaky wheel gets the grease.

Checklist: Managing the Referral Process

MANAGING THE REFERRAL PROCESS

1

What is the referral process?

Your doctor, a primary care physician, is submitting a referral request on your behalf for a specialist visit or other service. Your doctor belongs to a medical group which reviews the referral request to be sure that:

- You are referred to the most appropriate specialist or service
- The cost of your specialist visit or service is covered by your insurance
- You are treated promptly.

2

What happens when my doctor submits a referral?

- If your condition is an emergency, your doctor calls for immediate authorization.
- If your condition is *not* an emergency, your doctor sends the referral request to his/her medical group for review.
- The referral request and benefits review may take up to three (3) working days for non-emergencies.
- Your doctor will contact you to let you know the next step.

3

Important information regarding your referral request

Keep the following information on hand until your referral request is complete:

Referral #_____ Today's Date _____

Referring Doctor's Name_____

Referring Doctor's Office Telephone Number _____

If you don't hear from your doctor_____, contact your doctor's office
at the number above.   *date*

Medical Group Member Services Telephone Number _____

Specialist or Service Provider Name (if applicable) _____

Special instructions from your doctor _____

_____

_____

A CONSUMER TOOL FROM CALIFORNIA HEALTH DECISIONS

What to Do When You Have Problems with Your Health Plan

Whenever you have a problem with your health plan, be assertive. Don't think of any statement or decision from the plan as final, but rather as the beginning of a process. Many people who hear "no" from their plan will accept that as the final word. They may be unhappy, even bitter—but they give up. You won't, recognizing that if you push forward you'll get the right care. As we like to say about health care (and life), there isn't such a thing as "no," only "not yet."

Here's where knowledge of your rights will come in handy. What if your health plan takes several months to reimburse you for an expense? In New York State, there is a prompt payment law that mandates health plans reimburse you within 45 days. If they don't, they can be fined. There is even a hotline number to call if you find yourself in that situation.

What if your health plan tells you that a procedure or treatment is not covered? Ask them to show you exactly where in your member handbook it says the treatment is excluded. If there is not specific wording excluding it, then you have a good basis for appeal.

What if your health plan won't pay for the services you need, even after you complain? More than 30 states mandate "external appeals," giving you the right to appeal some types of managed-care decisions to an independent reviewer. Approximately half of people win these external appeals.

In addition to relying on friends and family, use the patient advocates in your community. For instance, if one of your family members is diagnosed with multiple sclerosis and your health plan is not providing appropriate services, call an office of the National Multiple Sclerosis Society or another MS organization. People working in these organizations have dealt with similar situations before, and can offer you good guidance.

If you get coverage through work, go to your friends in the employee benefits department. Businesses have begun paying more attention to the medical quality provided to their employees. Increasingly, businesses feel that the same sort of "Best Practices" that they use to run their businesses should be adopted by external contractors like benefits providers. Since individual workers have not taken the lead in demanding the top quality in medical services, employers are making it their job to do so.

Some of the nation's largest corporations, including General Electric and General Motors, have formed an organization called The Leapfrog Group to battle against medical errors and to guide their workers to the safest hospitals. If your company is not part of this effort, try to get them involved. (Contact the Business Roundtable, which is listed in Appendix A.) Your company should want to adopt the "Best Business Practices" for employee medical care used by the top U.S. companies.

Sample Letter: Appeal for Services Denied as "Not Medically Necessary"

[Date]
[Your Medical Group OR Health Plan]
Customer Service Department
[address]
RE: Appeal for [your name] OR URGENT APPEAL
    for [your name]
Subscriber # [your number]

Dear Customer Service Department:
    I am writing to appeal [name of medical group OR health plan]'s decision to deny authorization for [name of service, procedure OR treatment sought] for me. The [medical group OR health plan] has denied coverage for [name of

service, procedure OR treatment], as not medically necessary. I believe [name of service, procedure OR treatment
sought] is medically necessary to [treat or diagnose OR
address] my medical condition and is covered by my health
plan. [Name of medical group OR health plan] should
approve [name of service, procedure OR treatment] in my
case.

FAILURE TO PROVIDE IMMEDIATE TREATMENT
FOR MY CONDITION INVOLVES AN IMMINENT AND
SERIOUS THREAT TO MY HEALTH. I AM, THERE-
FORE, REQUESTING AN EXPEDITED REVIEW OF MY
APPEAL. PLEASE NOTIFY ME OF YOUR DECISION AS
SOON AS POSSIBLE, AND NO LATER THAN FIVE
DAYS [or time specified in your evidence of coverage]
FROM THE DATE OF MY REQUEST.

[Name of health plan] covers medically necessary services that are not specifically excluded. [Name of health
plan]'s definition of medical necessity is found on page [page
#] of my [Evidence of Coverage OR Summary Plan
Description]. Medical necessity is defined as:

[insert plan definition of medical necessity from your
member handbook]

As explained below, [name of service, procedure OR
treatment sought], for addressing my condition, falls within
this definition. The plan excludes treatments and procedures
listed on page [page #] of my [Evidence of Coverage OR
Summary Plan Description]. [Name of service, procedure
OR treatment sought] is not listed as an exclusion or limita-
tion under my health plan coverage.

[Name of service, procedure OR treatment sought] is
recommended for my condition by [name of doctor or specialist supporting your request]. Further, [the service, procedure OR treatment] is within the standards of good clinical
practice. {If you are in a state that has "mandated benefit
laws," or laws that require plans to provide certain coverage,

it can be helpful to refer to provisions that mandate coverage for the treatment or service you are seeking. The following language may be appropriate if there are "mandated benefits laws" that apply to your situation. The [medical group OR health plan]'s failure to provide [name of service, procedure OR treatment sought] also violates [California OR other] law which requires [applicable legal requirement]. (See Cal. Health & Safety Code § [code section number].)}

{In one or more paragraphs, describe your condition. Keep your description brief but sufficiently detailed to include a chronology of your symptoms, and any tests and treatments you have undergone. The amount of detail you use will depend upon your specific situation. Following is a sample paragraph.}

I have [name of condition OR "an undiagnosed condition"] and it affects my ability to conduct activities of daily living. I have previously received [types of other treatments you have tried, or diagnostic tests you have undergone, if any] to [treat AND/OR diagnose] my condition. However, my health problems have not been resolved. Without [name of procedure OR treatment], I will continue to experience [symptoms OR problems]. If left [untreated OR undiagnosed], my condition may require even more complex and costly treatment in the future.

I have included documentation of my medical condition, and information supporting the medical necessity of [name of service OR procedure], with this letter. Please let me know if any additional information will be helpful to my request. I can be reached at [**telephone number**].

Thank you for your immediate attention to this matter.

Sincerely,
*[**your name**]*
cc: {Possible individuals and/or groups to whom you can consider sending copies of your letter:}

[Health Plan Medical Director]
[Medical Group Medical Director]
[Your primary care physician]
[Your specialist]
[Your employer or insurance broker]
[Your state regulatory agency]

Attachments: {Material and documentation you can consider attaching:}

Copies of portions of plan member handbook or EOC stating coverage terms, (i.e. specific coverage provisions, and/or definition of medical necessity and list of exclusions and limitations);

Copy of referral;

Copy of letter from doctor (supporting treatment and supporting need for expedited review, if applicable);

Medical records;

Medical journal articles supporting medical necessity of care sought.

© 1999 Center for Health Care Rights, Los Angeles. Reprinted with permission.

Why UCR Is a Dirty Word

You may never have heard of UCR, but you will. UCR stands for Usual, Customary, and Reasonable. If you are in a PPO, POS, or any health plan where you can go "out of network" to see a doctor who is not on the preferred list, you must understand how the process works.

When you choose a health plan, you contractually accept its rules and regulations. A common rule is that going to an "in-network" doctor is less expensive. That's because the plan has previously negotiated set rates with the doctors. If you go to an "out-of-network" doctor, your cost will be higher.

Many people just assume that they can go to any "out-of-network" doctor in the area and their plan will pay 80% of the bill. But in most cases, your plan pays 80% of the amount it designates as its Usual, Customary, and Reasonable rate for that visit or procedure in that geographic area. The plan will reimburse you according to its own "fee schedule" for its usual and customary rate. You will have to pay any difference, and that difference can be a huge cost to you.

For instance, if you see an out-of-network doctor who charges you $200 for an office visit, but your plan's UCR fee is only $100, then a likely scenario is that the plan will only pay 80% of its UCR, for a total of $80. You will have to pay not only the remaining 20%, or $20, but the entire difference between the UCR and the total bill, or $100. You actually wind up paying $120—so you pay more than your plan pays.

Imagine that you don't discover all this until after you have seen that doctor several times. A lot of people go into a state of shock when they receive the first statement and see how much they are paying out of pocket.

UCR is sometimes called "Balanced Billing," although we don't see much that's balanced about it. We think that UCR should stand for Usually the Consumer is Ruined.

Here's how to avoid getting stuck in UCR hell: Before going to an out-of-network doctor, call the office manager in the doctor's office to find out what the fees are. Then call your health plan and ask for its UCR rate for that type of doctor visit for that condition in that geographic area. Be as specific as possible. It may not be easy to get the information, because health plans are often reluctant to tell you the UCR dollar amounts—putting patients in a Catch-22 situation. Sometimes they won't even tell doctors what the UCR amounts are!

If you are getting the runaround from your health plan, tell them outright that you are afraid you won't be able to afford the bills and have to know what your legal liability will be. The word "legal" may get their attention.

If your treatment includes a hospital visit, you may hear the term DRG. That stands for Diagnosis Related Group, which is part of a system of hundreds of different diagnoses for which doctors are reimbursed. If you are ready to be really assertive, ask your doctor for the DRG codes and read them off to the health plan customer service.

Once you know the UCR fee, go back to the out-of-network doctor's office and say that this is the dollar amount you have to work with. Be honest. Tell them that you know the UCR fee is probably less than what she normally receives and that you cannot afford much out-of-pocket cost, but that you really want to see this doctor. This presents the doctor with straightforward information. It appeals to her conscience in that you are trying to get the best care, and appeals to her ego in that you really want to see her.

"Loyalty counts," one doctor told us. "Most times special arrangements or fee structures can be worked out."

Doctor's fees can be negotiated, but you want to always do the negotiating ahead of time. The more information you have at the start, the better bargaining position you will find yourself in.

Why COBRA Is Worth It

COBRA stands for Consolidated Omnibus Budget Reconciliation Act, a federal law that was put into effect in 1986. Under COBRA, you are entitled to at least 18 months of continued health coverage when you leave a job with such benefits at a business with more than 20 employees. You are also eligible for extended coverage if your hours at work are reduced so that you no longer qualify for coverage. To receive coverage, though, you will have to pay 102% of the full premium during the 18 months.

Special rules extend COBRA, sometimes at a higher premium, for those who lose coverage through the death of a spouse or parent, divorce, and total disability. Many states have continuation laws for smaller companies with fewer than 20 employees.

Some of the details are complicated, but the important point is this: If you're going into a situation where you won't have health coverage, then sign up for COBRA. It's probably the best deal you'll find.

COBRA ensures that you will be able to stay in the same health plan. If your former employer switches plans, though, you will as well. You will pay more, because your employer no longer chips in and you're now paying the full cost—but the amount is still likely to be less than you will pay elsewhere.

It is your old employer's legal obligation to notify you of your COBRA rights. From the time of notification, you have 60 days to sign up, and then another 45 days to pay the premium—which gives you a good amount of flexibility. The 60 days only starts on the date of notification.

This continuity of coverage (being continuously covered without any gaps) is important, if only because of possible future exclusions for pre-existing conditions. Many employers don't explain it well because they don't see it as part of their job to help ex-employees. Make sure that you understand all of your options.

If you're leaving a job where you had health benefits to go to a job where you don't, COBRA is a great thing to have. It's also useful as a "bridge" until you become eligible for health benefits with a new employer. At many jobs, you are not eligible for health coverage until you have been employed for three months or more. COBRA bridges that gap.

Did you know that you can negotiate with your new employer about paying your COBRA monthly premiums? We know people who have done this and saved a lot of money. In a tight job market, this is a great money-saving perk that many people can negotiate. Some states also have programs to help people pay COBRA premiums.

Before leaving your old job, discuss COBRA in detail with your employee benefits people. Once you're on COBRA, your coverage may be administered by a third party that doesn't know what benefits you are entitled to receive. The third-party administrator may mistakenly deny coverage or reimbursements. If this ever happens, appeal vigorously. Under COBRA, your plan benefits stay the same.

When you exhaust COBRA, you fall under HIPAA—the Health Insurance Portability and Accountability Act. This federal law sets rules regarding portability, open enrollment in groups, noncancellation of individual policies, and the like. Some people have discovered that the coverage they were able to obtain under HIPAA was very expensive. Try to find another health plan before your COBRA coverage expires.

3.

How to Get the Best Care from Doctors and Other Practitioners

How to Choose a Doctor from a List

CHOOSING A DOCTOR CAN BE CONFUSING. THESE DAYS, many of us are simply handed a long list of doctors and told to make a decision. How do you make an intelligent selection from a list?

Some people have creative solutions. We know one man who simply looks for the most Jewish name on the list and makes the decision accordingly ("Irving Shapiro, M.D., is a good choice"). He's Jewish, so he can say that.

One health benefits expert told us that when people choose a doctor from a list, they focus on two things: which doctor is nearest to me, and which doctor has a name that I can pronounce? Understandable factors, yes, but we suggest that you do a little more research to ensure that you will get good care. Doctors are like any other professionals: some are excellent, most are pretty good, and some are no good. You want to find not only a good doctor, but the one who is best for you.

Ask as many co-workers, friends, and relatives as possible about their doctors. If you get health coverage through work, then your colleagues are an excellent source of referrals. Ask them who is good and who should be avoided. Find someone whose opinion you respect and who has a similar lifestyle to yours, and then consider using her doctor.

In addition to asking co-workers and friends who are in the same plan, you can request more information from the plan itself. Many plans now provide material on doctors' specialties, education, fees, office hours, languages spoken, and other information. Ask your plan what additional information it can provide to help you make a good choice.

Some plans have heard complaints about the difficulty of choosing a doctor from a list and have devised interesting tools. When Paul needed to choose a doctor from a list a few years ago, he got a pleasant surprise: "I've been in HMOs for most of my adult life, and I've chosen several doctors from lists. The last time I needed to choose a doctor from a list, I asked the HMO to send me more information. It mailed me 'baseball cards' with the doctors' photos, educational backgrounds, and even hobbies. I found this material helpful, and I felt better about making my decision."

When you have narrowed down the choice to two or three doctors, do more research. Find out where they went to medical school and did their internships and residencies, how long they have been practicing, and what professional associations they are affiliated with.

For basic information, go to your local library and ask for the *Directory of Board Certified American Medical Specialists*, which has information on more than half of all practicing physicians. You can also use AMA Physician Select, from the American Medical Association, at www.ama-assn.org.

Some forward-looking health plans and business groups have begun distributing information about how different medical practices rank on a variety of factors. PacifiCare, a large managed care company in California, is a leader in this regard. You can call to ask for its Quality Index, or visit its web site at www.pacificare.com. An employer association called the

Pacific Business Group on Health has similar information about West Coast doctor groups on its web site, www.healthscope.org. At least one forward-looking state, Massachusetts, is giving consumers more information about specific doctors. Massachusetts residents can get a "report card" on up to 10 doctors mailed or faxed to them. In addition to material on hospital accreditations and education, the report card contains information on disciplinary actions and malpractice cases. For more information, call (617) 727-0773 or go to www.massmedboard.org. We hope that other states will follow the lead of Massachusetts, but know that doctors' medical associations will fight against the adoption of similar programs.

Make sure that your doctor is board certified, meaning that he has completed rigorous training in his specialty. Approximately two-thirds of doctors are board certified, so you can consider this a reasonable standard of professionalism. For more information, contact the American Board of Medical Specialties at (800) 776-2378 or www.certifieddoctor.org.

A good credential is serving on the faculty of a teaching hospital. To become a faculty member, a doctor has to earn the respect and admiration of her peers. Hospitals are careful about the people they select as faculty members because they want to enhance their reputations while avoiding doctors who might expose them to legal liability (malpractice suits).

If you want to be treated at a specific hospital, then make sure your doctor has "admitting privileges" at that hospital. Otherwise, you are much less likely to receive care there. One hospital expert told us, "The most important thing to do is find out where your doctor has admitting privileges, because if you have to be admitted to a hospital, that's where you're going to wind up. That's also the place your doctor will send you for specialists. So know up front what hospitals your doctor is affiliated with."

If you have a relationship with a specialist that you want to continue, talk to that doctor before choosing a primary care physician. Deborah Kelly, a group benefits administrator in New York City, says, "I often tell people to 'work backwards.' A lot of consumers are set on which specialists they use, but are flexible on a primary care physician. I tell them to call the specialist's office and speak to the nurse, receptionist, or doctor—depending on their relationship. Ask them to recommend a primary care physician who works closely with the specialist's office. Referrals become *much* easier to get this way."

Kelly also puts in a word for talking to nurses, saying, "I found my great ob/gyn by asking the nurse at my son's pediatrician's office for a recommendation. Nurses are a great resource."

We recommend that you find a doctor who you like. A doctor could turn out to be a very important person in your life, so it's not superficial to want to like your doctor. The two of you will have a relationship, and like any good relationship, it should consist of communication and caring.

Compatibility matters. Studies of Massachusetts patients and Medicare beneficiaries have shown that patients get better care when they get along well and communicate smoothly with their primary care physician. When people understand their care, they are more likely to follow their treatment plans and get better. This has been demonstrated in studies of people with diseases ranging from high blood pressure and diabetes to ulcers and arthritis.

A study at Massachusetts General Hospital showed the importance of doctor-patient communication. Patients about to undergo surgery were visited the night before by an anesthesiologist. Half of the patients were given short, clinical descriptions of what would happen during their surgery. The other half were given long, sympathetic chats about what to expect after surgery and were assured that their pain would be taken care of. When the results were tabulated, those who had received the sympathetic chats were discharged from the hospital 2.6 days earlier than the others.

Dana Gelb Safran, Sc.D., of the New England Medical Center's Health Institute has done extensive research into effective doctor-patient communication. She recommends: "You want a doctor you trust, and who communicates with you effectively. You want a doctor who knows you as a person, and knows what your daily life is like. Find a doctor who knows you well enough that when they give advice, you feel comfortable following it."

A patient who feels that her doctor really cares about her as a human being is much more likely to follow that doctor's advice and get better. One study found that "adherence rates" of patients with strong connections to their doctors were more than double those of patients with weak relationships. Medical researchers say that doctors who take the time to learn about their patients gain "whole person knowledge." We think that's a great way to phrase it.

Researcher Dr. Sherrie Kaplan notes that most doctors are open to participatory decision making with their patients. "Participatory decision making works," she says. "It's positively correlated with better outcomes." That participation is a two-way street. Patients need to speak just as much as they want their doctors to listen. Passive patients, especially those with chronic conditions, don't do as well over time.

Some doctors describe finding the fit with patients as akin to a marriage. They recognize that the doctor-patient relationship is an important dynamic in the quality of care. And even though some doctors fail at it, most recognize that being personable is part of the job. In fact, there's an old saying among doctors that patients are more interested in Accessibility and Affability than they are in Ability.

The bottom line is this: If you and your doctor get along well and communicate better, ultimately you will get better care.

Don't get us wrong, ability matters greatly. But it's difficult for a patient to evaluate a doctor's ability, and the medical profession has blocked the collection and dissemination of objective measures of an individual doctor's skills. Because you will not be able to find out which doctors have the best objective records of treating patients, listen carefully to comments about doctors from friends and neighbors. If they express reservations not just about a doctor's personality or the office's efficiency, but suggest that anything less than good and thorough care was provided, that's a big red flag.

Did you know that you can interview prospective doctors? If you've narrowed down the list to a few choices, then why not call up each doctor's office and say, "I need to choose a doctor and I'm considering going with yours. I would like to arrange a time to speak with the doctor, either in person or over the phone, to see if she would be a good match for me. Can we set that time now?" Let the doctor's office choose whether to make it an office visit or a phone visit, because some doctors have strong preferences either way.

If it's a phone interview, don't ask for more than five minutes, because most doctors really are busy. Five minutes is a reasonable amount of time to request, and in that time, you should get a sense of what the doctor is like and whether you'll be compatible.

If you never get a five-minute appointment, then right away you know that the physician is not responsive. Do you really want to depend on someone like that? It also tells you that the doctor doesn't need your business. You want to find a doctor who wants your business.

Choose a doctor for yourself with as much care as you would for a family member who became seriously ill. As one woman told us, "All the mothers I know interview pediatricians carefully." If you can do it for your kids, you can do it for yourself.

You might also want to drop by the doctor's office, just to

see how it looks. How many people are in the waiting room? Is the staff pleasant? Does the office look well maintained, clean, and computerized? (Do they have any good magazines?) If you walk in and feel turned off right away, then this is probably not the place for you.

Sample Questions: Interview a Doctor

Have some questions written down before you interview the doctor. You don't want to ask just one question and then let the doctor go on for five minutes without interacting with you. Here are sample questions:

- How do you treat people like me who have *x* condition/needs/lifestyle?
- How can I reach you if *x* happens?
- Who treats your patients when you're away?
- When I come in for a visit, will I see you, or will I be handed off to another doctor?
- How long have you been in practice?
- Where did you go to medical school? What was your class standing?
- Where did you do your internship and residency?
- Are you board certified? Did you complete a fellowship?
- If I have an appointment about something serious, can I bring my spouse or close friend into the room with me?
- I like to bring written questions to an appointment so that I don't forget anything. How do you feel about this?
- Do you have any testimonials from patients?
- How much time do you spend with an average patient?
- If I have a problem that's beyond the scope of your training, will you refer me to a specialist? How does that work? Is it easy to get referrals?

After talking to a doctor for five minutes, you will almost certainly know if there's a good match. You will also have demonstrated clearly to the doctor that you're an educated patient.

If You Can Choose Any Doctor

If you're fortunate enough to be able to choose any doctor, then broaden your search. Talk to anyone you can find who is dealing with a health situation or condition similar to yours. The Internet is an excellent source of information and personal connections. You may also want to look up the Best Doctors lists that we mention below.

If you have just been diagnosed with a disease or chronic condition, you will probably be looking for a specialist. There are more specialists than primary care physicians, and finding the right one can be intimidating. You may be tempted to go with the first doctor suggested to you. As with any decision, the first choice may not be the best one. Also remember that if your primary care physician recommends a specialist, the suggestion could be based as much on his professional or personal affiliations as on the quality of the specialist. You want the best specialist, not your doctor's golfing buddy.

Diane Robertson of the not-for-profit group ECRI says that for patients, "one of the biggest problems is interpreting all the information—particularly when there are conflicting opinions among doctors about what works. Ask about your clinicians' experience and find out about their vested interests and their statistics."

Don't let yourself be rushed. Breast cancer survivor Jeanne Sather notes, "At the office where I had my mammogram done, they had me scheduled for a mastectomy before I even decided to have one." She wound up going elsewhere, and recommends, "If you're diagnosed, you may have weeks or months to get second or third opinions. It's important not to feel pressured."

Ask a specialist how many times he has performed this

exact procedure. You want to hear that the doctor has done hundreds or thousands of the procedure, not a few dozen. Every doctor needs to have a first patient—but don't let it be you.

The fact that experience counts among doctors is proven by the reports we discussed in Chapter One that documented mortality rates for coronary bypass operations in New York State. In 1996, the surgeons with the worst mortality rates had all performed less than 300 operations during the year. The surgeons with the best records had all performed more than 500.

If you're facing extensive treatment, ask about fees up front. You particularly want to know about the relationship between your health insurer and prospective doctors.

Here are some good resources for finding doctors:

- Best Doctors in America provides reference books and fee-based telephone counseling for individuals with critical or complex cases. For more information, call (888) DOC-TORS or go to www.bestdoctors.com.

- Castle Connolly Medical, Ltd., publishes thick Best Doctors books for the metropolitan areas of New York, San Francisco, and Los Angeles. These books are reasonably priced and are available in bookstores. For more information, call (800) 399-DOCS.

- Check "Best Doctors" articles in local magazines and newspapers.

- Several web sites now include information about individual doctors throughout the nation, including www.healthgrades.com and www.thehealthpages.com (free information) and www.askmedi.com and www.guidetotopdoctors.org (fee-based information).

- If you want a doctor affiliated with a specific hospital, call that hospital's switchboard and request the telephone number of its Physician Referral Service.

Help Your Doctor Help You

Time is precious with health professionals, so make things easier by going into an appointment ready for business. As the Boy Scouts say, be prepared.

Expert David Lansky suggests doing enough research that you understand the "standards of care" for your condition and the "benchmarks" for treatment. Not long ago this would have been beyond the capability of most people. But with the amount of information now available on the Internet and at local libraries, you can get a good sense of treatment options before you walk into a doctor's office. Several doctors have told us about seeing patients who come in with a printout of a study they found on the Internet—before the doctor has heard of the study. There are literally tens of thousands of articles published in medical journals every year, and no doctor can read every one. For a list of good web sites, see the section "Free Resources on the Internet" in Chapter Six.

You should prepare for a doctor's appointment like you would for a business meeting. After all, your next doctor's appointment is probably more important to you than your next office meeting. Be ready to ask specific questions, for instance, about experimental treatments or adverse drug interactions. Be honest if you have taken herbs as medicine or megadoses of vitamins without first consulting the doctor, or if you have not followed your treatment regimen.

Here's a helpful hint from expert Ellen Severoni: "Most individual treatment decisions are made at the level of the doctor or medical clinic. So understand the process. Become more savvy about how your doctor works." What kind of office does your doctor have? Is it a solo practice? An Individual Practice Association (IPA)?

What should you expect from your primary care doctor? According to the Institute of Medicine, primary care is "the provision of integrated, accessible health care services by clinicians who are accountable for addressing a large majority of personal health care needs, developing a sustained partnership with patients, and practicing in the context of family and the community."

Experts say that the quality of your relationship with a primary care doctor can be evaluated by looking at the following seven factors. How do you feel your doctor is doing on these seven points? Are there ways you can improve the doctor-patient relationship in any of these areas?

1. Accessibility of care
2. Continuity of care
3. Comprehensiveness of care
4. Clinical interaction, with thorough exams and good communication
5. Coordination, with your doctor making sure you get the right care
6. Humane interpersonal treatment, with a "whole person" orientation
7. A sustained partnership between doctor and patient, based on trust

7 Minutes with Your Doctor: How to Get the Most Out of a Doctor Visit

You've picked an excellent doctor. You're ready for your appointment. Now you must deal with managed care's biggest symptom: rushed doctors. The average length of time for a doctor's appointment is reported to be between 10 and 15 minutes, though several doctors have told us that they now have only seven minutes to spend per patient. As managed care pressures doctors to see more patients, visits keep getting shorter.

A 1995 survey found that 40% of doctors said they had cut back on the time they spent with patients during the previous three years. The situation has gotten so bad that some people refer to it as "hit and run medicine."

Even beyond time limitations, some doctors do not pay enough attention to patients. A study that appeared in the *Journal of the American Medical Association* in 1999 found that doctors often fail to listen to patients and that they make 91% of care decisions themselves, without any patient input. "Primary-care physicians frequently made decisions without discussing the intervention with the patient or seeking their involvement," wrote Clarence H. Braddock III, M.D. "These findings suggest that the ethical model of informed decision-making is not routinely applied in office practice."

So how can you make the most of those seven minutes while also getting your doctor to hear what you say?

Dr. Sherrie Kaplan, who has conducted a great deal of research into doctor-patient communication, recommends four overarching principles:

1. Prepare ahead of time.
2. Get ready to listen.
3. Stay focused on what the doctor is saying.
4. Ask questions.

You might think that people would routinely ask questions at a medical appointment, but Dr. Kaplan points out that many people don't—especially men. Studies have found that the question most commonly asked of medical personnel is "Where's the bathroom?" When they are sitting in an examining room "nervous and naked," patients can easily start to feel foolish and forgetful. Some patients don't even bring up the real reason for coming in until the end of the visit, as several frustrated doctors have told us.

That's why we suggest that you go into your doctor's office

well prepared. If you have a copy of your own medical record, bring it along in case the doctor's office can't find its own. (We'll tell you how to keep your own medical record in Chapter Five.) Bring your appointment book in case you need to schedule a follow-up visit or test. Come with a list of questions, along with pens and paper. Ask the most important questions first, and understand that the doctor may not have time to answer every single question. ("We've seen people come in with really long lists," one doctor told us with a sigh. Another doctor said that five questions should be the maximum.) The same is true of articles you've clipped out of newspapers and printed off the Internet—they can be a useful addition to the visit, but your doctor won't have time to read through every article and discuss its authenticity or relevance to your case.

Doctors use a system called HEAD for office visits. HEAD stands for History, Exam, Assessment, and Decision. Using the system, a doctor asks you questions about your medical history and current problems, examines you to see how the problems are affecting your body, assesses underlying causes and possible courses of actions, and then decides on the best approach to treating and solving the problem. Understanding that your doctor is proceeding in this order will help you get the most out of an office visit.

A visit to the doctor can be stressful, and many people forget a lot of what the doctor said as soon as they walk out the door. You can bring someone into the office to act as "a second pair of ears." More and more offices are open to having a loved one in the room. If you get a serious diagnosis, you may only hear part of it, so there is value in someone else being there.

One patient advocate told us about her own experience being diagnosed with a life-threatening illness. She said, "It was a good thing my husband was in there, because we were so shocked that neither of us heard everything the doctor said. But I absorbed about half of it, and my husband got most of the other half, so later on we were able to talk and piece together what was said."

What if no one is available to come to the appointment with you? Ask the doctor if you can tape-record the visit. Let your doctor know that you're making the tape so that you can better follow up on the doctor's suggestions. Because of fears about litigation, doctors may be wary of tape recorders. You can say, "This tape is just for my use, to make sure that I'm complying with the course of treatment."

If you're concerned that you won't have enough time with your doctor, simply ask her at the beginning of the appointment, "How much time do we have together? Because I have some important questions." Make eye contact with your doctor whenever possible.

If your doctor speaks too fast, don't feel bad about asking her to slow down. If she uses medical jargon you don't understand, ask for it in plain English. If you take notes and hear a word that's new to you, ask for the spelling. This tells the doctor that you need an explanation. It also gives you something to look up later. You can also ask the doctor to write the words down in your notebook, especially when they involve medical terms or pharmaceutical drugs.

Still not sure you get what the doctor is saying? Try rephrasing it. Tell the doctor, "I just want to make sure I'm understanding you. What you're saying is that . . . " Putting it in your own words will allow you to get a better grasp of the medical concepts, and will enable the doctor to see your perspective.

If you take several different prescription drugs, carry the containers with you to your initial visit, so the doctor can check for possible adverse interactions and make certain that you're taking the medicines correctly. Consider bringing your vitamins and herbs as well. You might want to prepare a list of your prescriptions and supplements to be added to your medical file.

If the doctor gives you a prescription form, make sure that you can read and understand it. The bad handwriting of doctors has always been a source of jokes, but it's a serious problem. People have died because pharmacists misunderstood a doctor's writing and gave the wrong prescription. Don't assume that your pharmacist is more of a handwriting expert than you are.

What if your doctor has her hand on the door and is about to leave the room? If you have more questions, you can just say, "I feel rushed, and I need more time to talk about this, because I'm feeling lousy and I need to know more." If the doctor cannot give you more time, ask for a *scheduled* time in the future for a follow-up telephone call. It's important that this time be scheduled on both of your calendars, or else it will be easy for the follow-up to slip through the cracks at the doctor's office. Make sure to "close the loop."

Using these techniques may make you stand apart from other patients. You will be asking for more time and attention than most, so ask with a good attitude and thank the doctor for explanations. If the doctor feels that she is being grilled, she might withdraw—as most people do when attacked. You want to be an assertive patient, but not a hostile one.

"You're a partner with your doctor," says prominent oncologist Morton Coleman, M.D. "Work together, because we all want the same goal: good care for you."

Why "Continuity of Care" Is Important and How You Can Get It

Another consequence of managed care is that people often find themselves seeing different primary care physicians within the same medical office. Many patients find themselves going to "their" doctor only to be seen by "some other" doctor. According to Dana Gelb Safran, Sc.D., "Many medical practices now prioritize access over continuity—so you can see a doctor, but not necessarily the same doctor. This happens because a lot of people want immediate access to care."

This clinic model doesn't work well for many people, especially seniors and those with chronic conditions. It's already hard enough to ensure continuity of care when employers change health plans frequently, much less when doctors pop in and out. HMOs are the most difficult to deal with on this front. The worst offenders are "Staff Model" HMOs that have their own offices. They have not generally recognized the importance of continuity of care.

People like seeing the same doctor over time and this continuity of care has been found to often mean better care. You want the best care, so we recommend that you get as much continuity of care as possible by choosing a good doctor and seeing her regularly. Realistically, there will be some times when your doctor is unavailable. Doctors get to take vacations like everyone else, and many physicians travel to medical conferences. But you should reasonably expect to see your doctor most of the time.

People in health care use the term "continuity of care," so you may want to use that term when you speak to them. We usually don't like health care industry jargon, but if it helps people get better care, let's use it.

If this sort of continuity is important to you, avoid joining a Staff Model HMO. You would be better off with an "IPA Model" HMO (where you visit doctors in their own offices), and best off in a health plan where you can choose your own doctor.

A study published in the *Archives of Internal Medicine* in January 2000 found that health plan executives believe "physicians practicing in open-model systems (ie, Fee-for-Service, POS, IPA/network-model HMOs) are inherently more concerned with establishing enduring patient relationships than physicians in closed-model systems (group- and staff-model HMOs). They noted that physicians in open-model systems knowingly assume responsibility for building and maintaining their patient panel as part of their professional life, while physicians in closed-model systems were said to largely rely on their plan to provide them with patients." To summarize: The greater control you have in choosing and changing doctors, the more likely that a doctor will work hard to keep your business.

Following is a checklist to help you get the most out of a visit to the doctor.

Checklist: Doctor's Visit

MEDICAL CHECKLIST

---

1 **Before you go to the doctor . . .**
- When you schedule your appointment, tell the office why you need to see the doctor.
- Make a list of questions (most important questions first), and things to talk about with your doctor, and take this with you to your next appointment.
- Ask your doctor what happens next in your treatment, and what you should do.
- Call your doctor for any test results 5-10 days after your visit.

2 **When calling your doctor, medical group or health plan . . .**
- Be prepared. Know what you want *before* you call.
- Find out whom you need to talk to. Is there a special coordinator to help you?
- Ask if the doctor, medical group or health plan needs any additional information to help you. Do they need additional information from:
  Your doctor_____ You _____ Other_____
- Ask when the issue will be resolved. *Date:* _____
- Ask who you should call if you have additional questions, or if the issue is not resolved to your satisfaction:
  Name:_____ Phone:_____
  If the issue is not solved on time, or you want to appeal a decision, call your medical group or health plan for more information.
- Notes: _____
  _____

3 **Important names, dates and phone numbers**
- Date and time of your call: _____
- Who did you talk to?
  Name:_____ Title:_____ Phone: _____
- If you need to call someone else, what is the name and phone number?
  Name:_____ Title:_____ Phone: _____

4 **Notes/things to do**
1. _____
2. _____
3. _____
4. _____

A CONSUMER TOOL FROM CALIFORNIA HEALTH DECISIONS

Sample Phone Call: When You Can't Get an Appointment with Your Doctor

What if you can't get even a seven-minute appointment with your doctor?

There are many "barriers" to health care, and we don't just mean cost and paperwork. Sometimes getting through to your doctor seems like a military maneuver. The phone systems are often not the greatest. And when you walk into a doctor's office, the nurses and receptionists and the desks and doors are there on purpose—to create barriers between you and the doctor.

If you can't get the appointment you want, be firm and assertive, but polite and reasoned, in order to get what you need:

Receptionist: Doctor's office.

You: Hello, this is _____, and I'm a patient of Dr. Jane Smith. I need to get an appointment with her tomorrow.

R: I'm sorry, the doctor is all booked up. I can fit you in next Friday.

Y: No, I need to see the doctor tomorrow. It's urgent. [Explain reason.]

R: Is this an emergency? If it's an emergency, you should go to the emergency room.

Y: It's urgent, but not an emergency.

R: We might be able to find another doctor to see you tomorrow. Let's see, Dr. Johnson might have an opening.

Y: *I need to see my doctor. She knows my history, and I need the continuity of care. [Use the medical terms.]*

R: *Dr. Johnson is very capable, and he'll have your chart.*

Y: *I've been seeing Dr. Smith for two years, and she knows my whole history. I saw her a few months ago, and told her I was worried about something, and now it's happening again. I need to see her.*

R: *I could ask her to call you.*

Y: *Can you put me through now?*

R: *No, she is unavailable now. Would you like to leave a message?*

Y: *No, I really need to see her tomorrow. [If you leave a message, it is uncertain when the doctor will receive it, how it will be written down, and when she will call you back, along with other variables.] I'm really not feeling well. I don't mind waiting a little if you could squeeze me in.*

R: *Well, I might be able to fit you in tomorrow around 11.*

Y: *Yes, that would be very good. Thank you for your help. I really appreciate it. [Once you have pushed for good service, recognize when you receive it and express your appreciation.]*

A Message Just for Doctors

We wrote this section especially for doctors, although we think that everyone can benefit from reading it.

First, we want to say that we greatly respect doctors. Julie is alive partly because of excellent doctors. Paul witnessed enormous dedication and skill among AIDS specialists.

We also understand that the last two decades have been difficult for many physicians. The past 20 years have brought the rise of managed care, the loss of prestige for many doctors, uncertainty about income, and increasing levels of frustration—not to mention real fears of litigation in our lawsuit-happy society.

We encourage patients at all times to work with their doctors, to talk to their doctors, to be informed patients, and to have respect for medical personnel.

However, we have noticed that some doctors are unwilling to listen to criticism of any doctor or of anything in the medical profession. In response, we must say, "Get over it." There are excellent doctors and poor doctors, just like in any profession.

We as a nation should not allow incompetent doctors to continue practicing, no matter how small a percentage of the whole they constitute. The medical profession has shown itself to be incapable of monitoring its own members. Recently New York State took action against a brain surgeon who was accused of operating on the wrong side of one of his patients' brains—for the second time in five years!

The white wall of silence that protects bad doctors and medical mistakes is just as wrong as the blue wall of silence that protects bad cops. Your political lobby, the AMA, has not served you well by fighting against common-sense consumer protections.

With the rise of the Internet, the growing number of pharmaceutical interventions and medical devices, and the increasing torrent of health information, the role of the doctor is destined to change in the future. We think that doctors will benefit by viewing themselves as teachers and partners to their "clients," rather than as infallible entities making decisions for passive patients. The "show up and shut up" attitude toward patients doesn't work any more.

Talking to your patients is good for you, the doctor. Doctors with more participatory styles get consistently better ratings from patients. Like it or not, patient ratings are an increasingly important tool for health plans.

Doctors also need to be more willing to discuss cost—the biggest concern of health consumers today. Many doctors have adopted the attitude that they cure people and others must sort out the bills. That doesn't cut it anymore. Recently Paul saw his doctor, who recommended a booster shot. The doctor said that Paul could get the shot there right away, but added that it might not be covered by insurance. Realizing that he didn't have much cash on him, Paul asked if the office took credit cards. The doctor replied, "I don't know." C'mon, Doc—you should know how your own front desk works!

We hope that doctors will listen to those prominent physicians who have stressed that there should be greater doctor-patient communication, that systems should be put into place to prevent medical mistakes and to report serious ones, and that all doctors should be retested and relicensed to make sure that they remain current on medical standards and best practices.

Most doctors are talented and dedicated professionals. We want you to thrive. But in the age of 100 channels and 10 million web sites, you will only do so in the clear light of day.

When to Fire Your Doctor

We are all consumers of health care, and we should all act that way. So if your doctor is not giving you good care, not returning your phone calls, and not being responsive to your needs, why are you putting up with it? Instead you should feel comfortable and satisfied with your doctor. Not only are you paying a lot of money for her services, but you need to have a good relationship so that you can get the best care.

You can fire your doctor. You are the customer. One area where consumers have a lot of flexibility—even in HMOs—is in choosing doctors. If you're not happy with your doctor, change! More than half of households have changed doctors during the past two years. There are more than 700,000 doctors in this country. There must be one in your area who is right for you.

You might want to give your doctor a last chance before going elsewhere. Just like you can call before choosing a doctor to ask for a five-minute interview, if you're unhappy, you can call and ask for a five-minute consultation. Say that you want to talk about your "medical needs, and how they are not being met." If your doctor or her staff won't agree to this, then it may well be time to move on. If she does listen, then this is your chance to calmly tell your doctor how you feel and to ask for a response. Perhaps the discussion will prompt a more positive course of action. If not, at least you'll know that you made the effort.

Then if you do need to hire a new doctor, you can go back to the beginning of this chapter, and start over wiser for the wear.

Alternative Health Care— More for Your Money?

What is alternative health care? One definition is "Interventions that are neither taught widely in medical schools nor generally available in U.S. hospitals." These therapies include acupuncture, chiropractic, magnets, prayer, herbal medicine, relaxation techniques, massage, spiritual healing, megavitamins, self-help, guided imagery, folk remedies, energy healing, homeopathy, hypnosis, and biofeedback.

Alternative care is often also called "complementary" or "integrative" care, which are considered to be more favorable terms by many practitioners.

However alternative these therapies may be, they are increasingly popular. More than 40% of American adults say that they have used alternative techniques, and there are now more annual visits to alternative practitioners than to medical doctors. We spend $4 billion a year on herbal remedies alone. Even bastions of the medical establishment like the *Journal of the American Medical Association* are examining alternative treatment. The journal declared that some methods are valuable for patients, while others have no merit.

One reason that alternative health care has become so popular is that its practitioners often give a great deal of compassion—and time. A prominent oncologist, himself an advocate of complementary care, puts it this way: "I'm very busy, so I spend an average of seven minutes with each patient. Even though I give very good care, a lot of people feel that's not enough time. But when my patients go to see an alternative practitioner, they usually get a full hour of that person's time. They get to sit and talk and discuss for sixty minutes—something that I could never give them." It's clear that many consumers feel they get better value from alternative care than from traditional medicine.

We believe that you should decide what's best for your own health, in consultation with medical professionals. If you use alternative care, speak with a doctor about potential conflicts between conventional and alternative techniques. Many people feel sheepish about discussing alternative therapies with their medical doctor, so they go into the "alternative closet." Refusing to discuss therapies with your doctor can cause problems though. For instance, some herbs can cause harmful interactions with prescription drugs. So can high doses of certain vitamins. Studies recently published in *The Lancet* found that St. John's wort, a popular herbal treatment for depression, can reduce the effectiveness of drugs taken by heart transplant patients and people living with HIV.

If you're going to have a surgical procedure, tell your doctor about any herbs you have been taking, in addition to vitamins and over-the-counter drugs. The American Society of Anesthesiologists has stated that popular herbs like ginseng, gingko biloba, and St. John's wort may affect blood pressure or heart rate during surgery. It recommends that you suspend taking herbs or alternative medicines two weeks before surgery.

There is far less standardization of alternative health products than of prescription drugs, so just because something is labeled "natural" doesn't mean that it's safe. Several investigative studies have found that herbal preparations sometimes contain far less of the active ingredient than is claimed on the label. For instance, a recent test of 13 brands of the popular herbal product Sam-e found that only seven had contents consistent with the label. All of the mislabeled brands had lower amounts of Sam-e—some far lower.

Be a discerning consumer. Similarly, check the qualifications of alternative practitioners before seeing them. These practitioners can range from highly-skilled professionals to individuals with little, if any, training.

A good source of information about alternative care is the National Institutes of Health's National Center for Complementary and Alternative Medicine Clearinghouse, which can be reached at (888) 644-6226 or nccam.nih.gov.

An often unstated part of controversies over alternative therapies is that some have a religious or spiritual aspect. There's no doubt that the power of belief is very strong. An example is the well-documented "placebo" effect. In almost any treatment, between one-third and two-thirds of patients show improvement just from being treated—even if they're receiving a sugar pill (placebo) that has no actual effect.

Most doctors recognize the power of belief. They also try to stay up-to-date on a wide range of medical topics. If you're a consumer of alternative therapies, continue to work with a medical doctor, too. Find one who will talk with you in a non-judgmental way.

Health plans are slowly beginning to cover some alternative treatments. ("Very slowly," one alternative care consumer told us.) Check with your plan for coverage details before you visit any practitioners.

When Not to Use Alternative Practitioners

There are times to stay away from alternative practitioners. In emergencies, go the closest emergency room. If you have a life-threatening illness, always see a medical doctor first. Your choices are your own, but we advise you to go with the most proven medical treatment before using alternative therapies.

Be suspicious of anyone who insists that you stop seeing any medical doctor or taking any prescription drug, or who describes conventional medicine in extreme terms, using words like "poison," "conspiracy," and "mind-control."

We have seen tragic cases of people with AIDS and cancer who stopped their treatments because someone convinced them that an alternative technique would completely cure them. They died. We have only contempt for con artists who play on the fears and hopes of desperately ill people by pushing snake oil and false promises.

How to Get the Most from Your Pharmacist

Pharmacists play an important role in this country's health care. People have a lot of respect for their pharmacists. In poll after poll, pharmacists are named one of the nation's most trusted professions.

Your pharmacist is a great source of information about the medications you're taking. Feel free to ask him lots of questions. Our experience is that pharmacists like talking to their customers and learning about their problems. Pharmacists can also play a key role in preventing improper medication interactions by keeping track of all of the drugs you're taking. Because herbs can cause dangerous interactions, tell your pharmacist about any herbs you have been taking as well.

Try to go into the pharmacy already knowing about your condition and the medication you will be receiving. For marketing reasons, pharmaceutical manufacturers are increasingly putting out new medications with names similar to existing drugs, creating confusion and the potential for mistakes in dispensing. If you know the name of the drug you're supposed to get, tell the pharmacist as you hand him the prescription slip. If you don't, and the pharmacist cannot read your doctor's handwriting (which happens more often than you think), be understanding while he calls your doctor for more information. If you have to wait to get an answer, even if it causes you inconvenience, that's far better than getting the wrong medication.

Because of the high cost of drugs, it can be tempting to fill one prescription at a drugstore and another prescription at a warehouse club and yet another over the Internet. If you use multiple sources, it's especially important that you tell each pharmacist about all of the drugs and herbs you take.

If you have problems with a medication, like side effects, talk to your doctor or pharmacist. More than 2 billion prescriptions are dispensed every year in this country—and two-thirds of people don't take the full course of drugs. Among seniors, one-fifth of hospitalizations are caused by failure to take medications or by adverse drug interactions. You may be tempted to stop taking a prescription when you feel better, or if the side effects become bothersome. Consult with a professional first to make sure it's safe to stop.

Finally, remember to throw away old prescription drugs. The Council on Family Health recommends that you go through your medicine cabinet once a year to clean out old medications. Flush them down the toilet so that they don't create poison hazards for children or pets. And always keep prescription drugs and vitamins in a cool, dry place, out of the reach of children.

4.

How to Get the Best Care in Hospitals

Choose a Hospital—and Choose the Best

WHY SHOULD PEOPLE CARE ABOUT WHICH HOSPITAL THEY select? After all, most people rush to whichever hospital is closest in an emergency, and travel to the hospital their doctors suggest for other procedures. They consider hospitals to be safe places where they will receive excellent care. Our nation has thousands of hospitals, though, and there are differences between hospitals. There are also risks in any hospitalization, no matter how minor the procedure.

The 1999 report from the Institute of Medicine about medical mistakes in hospitals has awakened many people to the importance of choosing the right facility and being a good consumer. That report—which found that up to 98,000 Americans each year are killed by medical mistakes in hospitals—is just the tip of the iceberg. We have all heard the frightening stories of how a hospital visit can go horribly wrong, including tragic cases of people who died while undergoing "routine outpatient surgery." One of the sources for the Institute of Medicine report was a 1991 study of New York State hospitals by the Harvard University School of Public Health which estimated that in the studied year (1984), 13,451 patients died of injuries caused by treatment, and 6,895 patients died as the result of negligent care—just in one state in one year.

A recent study found that 106,000 hospital patients die each year from adverse drug reactions, many caused by error. And then there are hospital-acquired infections. The Centers for Disease Control and Prevention estimates that "nosocomial," or hospital-acquired, infections kill nearly 90,000 patients each year. The most common infections are urinary tract infections, pneumonia, surgical site infections, and primary bloodstream infections. Nosocomial infections rates are 5 to 10 times higher in Intensive Care Units, which house the sickest patients, than in general wards.

Unwashed hands are a leading source of hospital-acquired infections, killing thousands each year—although it has been documented for more than a century that washing hands before touching patients saves lives. All doctors and nurses have been told for their entire careers that they must wash their hands before touching a patient, yet many violate this most basic safety procedure on a daily basis. In an especially tragic incident, bacteria from beneath the long fingernails of nurses have been linked to the deaths of eight babies in the intensive care unit of an Oklahoma City hospital.

Despite all of these problems, many hospitals are reducing their numbers of registered nurses and replacing them with "nursing aides" who have received little training.

We don't list these numbers to scare you but to reinforce the importance of choosing a good hospital and, once you are there, of being an informed and assertive patient. If you can be a "defensive driver" on the highway, you can be a "defensive patient" in the hospital. For instance, patients can and should tell doctors and nurses to wash their hands before touching them.

Hospitals need your business. Twenty-seven percent of hospitals lost money in 1998, and more than one-third of all hospital beds in this country are empty at any time. Some hospitals which should have closed their doors remain open primarily because of political pressures. Even if a hospital is little-needed, its community does not want it to close. Its employees are afraid of losing their jobs and the politicians representing its neighborhood can get votes by demanding that it stay open.

Meanwhile, some inner city and rural areas have too few hospitals. Until there is a shakeout among underperforming hospitals, or until we have the courage to create a national Hospital-Closing Commission modeled after the Military Base-Closing Commission, there will be more hospital beds than needed. And these hospitals will often be in the wrong places.

Because of the oversupply of hospital rooms, patients can use their purchasing power to get the best care. You don't have to just go to the hospital that your doctor suggests. A doctor often has "admitting privileges" at more than one hospital. If your doctor's choice of hospital is not your first choice, then take a little time to do your own research.

You can get a free report on any hospital from the Joint Commission on Accreditation of Healthcare Organizations (JCAHO), which accredits most U.S. hospitals. The JCAHO is not an unbiased organization. On the contrary, it gets most of its funding from hospitals, meaning that it has a built-in conflict of interest. Not surprisingly, it rates most hospitals extremely favorably, and very rarely denies accreditation to even poor-performing hospitals. Still, if you are considering a hospital, it's worth looking at its JCAHO report. If the report is anything less than laudatory, that's a warning sign. As one government official told us, "The JCAHO is such an easy grader, if you see anything less than excellent marks for a hospital, you know not to go there." To get a free JCAHO report, call (630) 792-5000 or go to www.jcaho.org.

Once you're in the hospital, be an active participant in your own care. Hospitals are set up to make patients feel passive and powerless, "nervous and naked." Don't buy into it.

"I usually advise people who are going into the hospital to

write down what happens to them every day," says Susan Dressler, CCAP, of the Alliance of Claims Assistance Professionals. "Really monitor your care. Participate in the situation."

Having friends and family around is particularly important when you're in the hospital, because you may be sedated or too ill to keep track of things yourself. Recruit your loved ones to be your eyes and ears, and to act as your personal patient advocates. Ask them to come in shifts so that you spend as little time alone as possible.

If you have problems in a hospital, confront the issues as soon as possible. Appeal quickly to the hospital's patient representatives and administration, who should be reachable through the phone in your room. The patient representatives are there to respond to consumer complaints and you should make full use of them. If they're not responding adequately, call the hospital's chief executive. You will probably not get a direct response, but the call itself may prompt better care.

Do not accept excuses. Be firm. You deserve excellent care and excellent service—and yes, you are paying for it.

Even if most of your hospital bill is being picked up by a health plan or government program, your tax dollars have gone into that hospital for decades. Year after year, through your health insurance premiums and taxes, you have been paying for their buildings, equipment, supplies, and salaries. And what about all of those community fund-raisers, charity committees, special events, and even bake sales you supported? Now the time has come for the hospital to give you the best care.

Many hospitals are technically not-for-profit, but a lot of people are making a lot of profit at these hospitals—including administrators, star doctors, pharmaceutical companies, and other businesses. Some large hospitals have annual revenues of close to a billion dollars, with CEOs and top physicians who make half a million to a million dollars a year. You may think this is a good thing, because it attracts top people to medicine and encourages innovation. Or you may think it's a bad thing, because it puts a profit mentality into life-and-death issues. Either way, the situation isn't likely to change any time soon.

We suggest that you think of yourself as a medical customer who deserves excellent care, service, and attention at all times—even when you're in your most vulnerable state. Especially then.

If you feel that you're being pushed out of the hospital too soon, have a friend or relative look up the average stay for your procedure. You can find guidelines that specify the appropriate hospitalization duration from the National Guideline Clearinghouse on its web site at www.guideline.org. You can also contact not-for-profit groups like the American Diabetes Association and American Heart Association, which have developed treatment protocols that are widely accepted.

In some cases, there are state or federal laws mandating minimum stays. For instance, the federal Newborns' and Mothers' Protection Act of 1996 says that most health plans cannot restrict benefits for a hospital stay in connection with childbirth to less than 48 hours following a vaginal delivery or 96 hours following a delivery by cesarean section. For Medicare beneficiaries, there are special rights of appeal for hospital stays.

On the other hand, if you feel that you're being kept in the hospital too long, you can check yourself out without a doctor's signature. This is called leaving Against Medical Advice (A.M.A.). You're not legally obligated to sign release forms, but we recommend that you talk to an outside patient advocate before leaving.

After the hospital stay, if you have problems with billing or other matters—and this is common—don't be shy about complaining to the hospital, your health plan and employer, local and state regulators, elected officials, and the news media.

We hope that you won't have to go to a hospital soon. However, if you do, we'd like your experience to be positive. If you're not so fortunate, don't sink into feeling sorry for yourself. Fight against the illnesses that threaten you, and fight against anything that stands in the way of your receiving quality care and service.

Why a "Big Name" Hospital Isn't Always the Best Choice for You

You want to find a hospital that's going to serve you the best, considering your preferences and specific conditions. As Julie notes, "I went to the 'best' cancer center in the country, but it certainly wasn't the best for me."

Julie was so disenchanted with the "top" cancer hospital in New York that she chose to get a bone marrow transplant at a hospital in Seattle. She found the Seattle facility to be far superior in patient care.

Heart disease is another area of treatment where we have seen discrepancies about what is "best." In our research, we found that some lesser-known hospitals that performed a high volume of heart surgery (Coronary Artery Bypass Graft Surgery and Angioplasty) had far better mortality rates than big, well-known hospitals that heavily advertised their heart centers. So which hospital would you rather pick?

Just because a hospital is well-known does not mean it will be best for you. If a hospital is renowned for treating lung disease and you're going to have a baby, you would do well to find out its reputation for childbirth and neonatal care. And just because a hospital is tops at doing research on a particular disease doesn't mean that you will get the best treatment there. Look for a center which focuses on patient care. That said, research institutions sometimes can offer treatments unavailable elsewhere. Breast cancer survivor Jeanne Sather says, "I went to a hospital that had a Breast Center. Everyone there saw me the same day, which sold me on them. And they offered me a procedure that no one else had."

At a teaching hospital, you may wind up getting poked and prodded by an array of medical students. You may also find yourself becoming an object of discussion on "rounds," where doctors talk about you in the third person as if you couldn't hear them. Be aware that you don't have to put up with it. You can opt out of these exams and discussions.

If you're going to be hospitalized for a relatively simple procedure (like normal delivery of a baby) or elective surgery, then a smaller hospital may be the appropriate choice. Many patients say that they get better care and more personal attention at small community hospitals than at large teaching hospitals.

If you're facing a rare or complicated surgery, however, you will probably want to take the opposite tack, traveling as far as you need to get the finest care at the very best institution. People are often afraid to travel to a different city for medical care, thinking, "I have to be close to my family and friends." So they go to the biggest local hospital and hope for the best. We recommend that you go wherever you must to get the best care. We recently heard from a woman who lives in the New York City area but always goes to Boston for medical care, because she thinks the standard of care is better there. We don't know if that's true, but if she feels that way, more power to her for making her own choices.

Most people don't seek out the best medical care because they're too intimidated by their illnesses—and by the health care system. But when you become an educated patient, you will make informed choices, and you will probably live longer and better as a result.

Medical Mistakes are Epidemic— What You Need to Know

As you learned earlier in this chapter, up to 98,000 Americans die every year from medical mistakes in hospitals. That's the finding of the Institute of Medicine, an arm of the National

Academy of Sciences, the nation's top scientific advisory group. More people die each year from medical mistakes than die from AIDS, breast cancer, prostate cancer, or even highway accidents!

A study in the Veterans Administration hospital system found not only a high level of mistakes, but that the mistakes were serious ones. It states that "the adverse events reported by the V.A. were so serious that twenty-four percent of the patients died. One in four died."

A study of Chicago hospital patients published in the medical journal *The Lancet* in 1997 found that medical mistakes occurred in 45% of patients. Of these, 18% experienced serious complications. For each day in the hospital, the patients' chances of being injured increased 6%.

These findings were no surprise to us, or to many people working in health care. There have been other reports with similar results, but the health care industry swept them under a rug and refused to do much about the problem. Because the latest reports got a lot of media attention, we hope major changes will come about. That won't be easy though. Even now, the American Medical Association is opposed to mandatory reporting of serious medical mistakes. Worse, some federal health officials have decided against pressing for mandatory reporting, putting themselves on the side of the medical industry rather than the general public.

There's virtually no oversight of hospitals today. It's one area where the public just "assumes" that there's effective oversight—wrongly. As noted earlier, the only national body that monitors hospitals, the JCAHO, receives most of its funding from the very hospitals it supposedly oversees, and it rarely denies accreditation to anyone. One former hospital administrator told us how the JCAHO gave hospitals advance notice of its inspections, allowing hospitals to cover up problems. She added, "Although they're supposed to be the accreditation team that goes out and does a white glove standard of care, these people are really embedded in the medical industry." In the rare cases where the JCAHO does deny accreditation to a hospital, it keeps the action secret, failing to inform the public about a dangerous institution.

If there were ever a good reason for being an assertive consumer of health care, medical mistakes is that reason. Fortunately, people are starting to get the message. In the wake of the Institute of Medicine report, we heard a few doctors grumbling that their patients were asking more questions. The doctors meant it as a criticism. We were thrilled to hear it.

During her four years of treatment, Julie had her own experiences with medical mistakes. One of the worst mistakes caused her a great deal of discomfort: "I had to spend two hours in surgery while doctors put an IV line into my neck. That night, while I was resting in my room, an attendant came in and started working on the IV lines. I heard a snip and asked him, 'What are you doing?' He said he was carrying out his instructions. It didn't sound right, but I figured he knew what he was doing, and I was really tired. Later I found out that he had mistakenly removed the same line that had been put in that day. So I had to spend another two hours in surgery! I wished that I had been more aggressive in demanding answers. After that experience, I was."

Contrary to popular belief, hospitals are not "safe" places where people can expect everything to go right. As long as human beings are in charge of medicine, there will be human error. Most medical mistakes are the result of human error, whether that's giving the wrong drug, operating on the wrong part of the body, or mixing up patient charts.

The answer is not to blame people for being fallible, but to install safety systems that catch medical mistakes before they can cause injury or death. Hospitals have been slow to install such systems. The Institute of Medicine report concluded that "health care is a decade or more behind other high-risk industries in its attention to ensuring basic safety."

Yet the hospital industry doesn't have to search far for safety models. The airline industry has been developing safety systems for decades, making sure that most human error is corrected before it can cause any harm. As a result, air travel is far safer now than it has ever been. Within the medical field, anesthesiologists undertook a significant effort to reduce medical errors and were remarkably successful.

Hospitals can cut down on medical errors by insisting that both a doctor and nurse are present when powerful drugs like cancer medications are administered to a patient. Other cutting-edge techniques involve using bar codes for medications and even patients (on hospital wristbands). One-third of hospitals now have computer systems where doctors can enter orders for drugs and tests, although most hospitals don't require their use and some doctors refuse to learn how they work.

If you go into a hospital, what can you do to protect yourself? It all goes back to being an informed consumer. A list of 10 steps to avoid becoming the victim of a medical mistake follows this section of the book. Ask the hospital's patient representative what steps the hospital takes to prevent mistakes, and notice if its caregivers are following the rules.

Realize that just because you're a hospital patient doesn't mean you have to be passive. We recently told a friend with health problems to make sure when he went into the hospital that all medical personnel washed their hands before touching him. His response was, "I can't do that! If I'm a hospital patient, I can't tell doctors and nurses what to do—they're the medical staff!" It was clear that he felt intimidated by the staff, which is understandable. But your life has to come first. Thousands of people die every year in hospitals because medical personnel don't wash their hands. If there's anything to not be intimidated about, it's protecting your own life.

Be especially vigilant with orderlies and nurse aides, who

may have received very little training before beginning their jobs. If you have concerns about safety that you're afraid to bring up with doctors and nurses, contact the hospital's patient representative immediately. Or have one of your relatives or friends raise the issue for you.

Another type of safety to consider is that of your belongings. Theft and other crimes are surprisingly common in hospitals, so don't bring valuables or expensive belongings with you. Personal items help to make a hospital stay more comfortable, but don't take along anything that's irreplaceable.

Even in a hospital, you can be an assertive patient. We heard a case study at one of our recent speaking engagements. An elderly man told us that during his hospitalizations he kept a notebook and wrote down everything that happened, including every pill he was given. The first time he was in the hospital he was viewed very suspiciously for this. The nurses treated him like a "problem patient." The second time he went into that hospital, he spoke with the head nurse at the beginning of his stay, and told her that he was making his notes because he kept his own records and wanted to have a log for his own safety. He found that he got much better treatment during the second visit. The head nurse would even stop by and ask how he was doing.

The moral of the story? Be informed. If you don't understand what's happening, ask. If a pill looks different from the other pills you have taken, ask why. You should always get a response.

Based on our own experiences in talking to health professionals, we suspect that the health care sector will continue to be slow to confront the issue of medical mistakes. In the manuscript of our first book, we included some very well-documented information about the number of people who are killed by medical mistakes. One government health official who read the manuscript wrote in the margin, "Are you sure this is right?"

10 Steps for Avoiding Becoming the Victim of a Medical Mistake

1. **Keep a notebook by your bed and write down what happens to you.** In effect, you are keeping your own chart. If you're not well enough to write everything, ask visitors to help. This notebook lets the staff know that you are vigilant. It also makes you an active participant in your own care. Ask whatever questions about your care that you think are appropriate.

2. **Insist that doctors, nurses, and attendants wash their hands or put on fresh gloves before they touch you.** If you don't feel up to it, put up the sign we printed on a following page, which says, "Please wash hands before touching the patient, following standard protocols." Also write your name in large letters on a piece of paper and put that above your bed so that a busy nurse doesn't give you a medicine or procedure intended for another patient.

3. **When you are given injections or pills, ask what they're for.** If you're given something that you've never seen before, ask why it's different. Most medications are given at the same time each day, so if something comes at a different time, ask why. You need to get the "right drug, right dose, right route, right time, for the right patient."

4. **If you're having surgery, make sure that the correct part of your body is marked ahead of time.** Try to have your surgery scheduled early in the day and early in the week, when you're most likely to receive continuity of care from doctors and nurses. Experts advise against having surgery on Friday afternoons, because you will be recovering during the weekend when few doctors are around in the event

you have complications. Ask which doctor will be on call while you're recuperating. If it's a doctor you've never met, ask to meet him before your surgery. If you're getting elective surgery, don't schedule it during the month of July. That's when the new interns are just arriving, fresh out of medical school and with limited hands-on experience.

5. **Before surgery, speak to the anesthesiologist as well as the surgeon.** Tell the anesthesiologist what conditions you have and what medications and herbs you take. Even mention how much alcohol you drink and whether you take any illegal drugs. Make sure that this anesthesiologist is the one who will be in the operating room, that he will be there for the entire length of the operation, and that he is board certified in anesthesiology.

6. **Have friends and relatives visit as often as possible** to check in, and to advocate for you when you don't feel well enough.

7. **Try to introduce yourself right away to the head nurse and patient representative.** That way, you'll know where to turn if you have concerns, and they'll know you as an individual rather than a room number.

8. **Be nice to the nurses!** They can make your stay a lot easier, especially if they feel empathy for you as a person rather than viewing you as just another patient. Ask your friends and family to be nice to them as well, and to consider bringing candy or flowers for the nurses' station.

9. **Be careful what you eat.** Pass on undercooked eggs or other undercooked food, which can contain harmful bacteria that could make you sick. Don't eat anything on the day before you have surgery. If you can't stand the hospital food, ask

your friends and relatives to bring you healthy food from outside. Ask the nurses to lend you delivery menus for nearby restaurants. (If you order food, buy something extra for the nurses and ask for two new delivery menus. Give one new menu back to the nurses and keep the other for yourself.)

10. **If you can afford a private room, get one.** You'll be less likely to become infected by a roommate or that patient's visitors, and you'll eliminate the risk of a nurse giving a medication to the "wrong patient in the right room." It will also be easier for you to rest.

Sample Sign: Please Wash Hands!

We give you permission to photocopy the sign we've created. Tape the copy up near the head of the bed where it can be seen easily.

Please wash hands before touching the patient, following standard protocols.

PATIENT NAME:_____

_____

_____

ALLERGIES:_____

_____

_____

"A Patient's Bill of Rights" in the Hospital

You have stated rights in the hospital. According to guidelines issued by the American Hospital Association, a hospital patient has the right to:

- Considerate and respectful care.
- Complete information about his/her treatment and condition in terms the patient can reasonably understand.
- Know the identity of physicians, nurses, and others involved in their care, as well as when those involved are students, residents, or other trainees.
- Information necessary to give informed consent prior to the start of any procedure or treatment.
- Refuse treatment and be informed of the consequences.
- Have an advance directive (such as a living will, health care proxy, or durable power of attorney) for health care.
- Privacy concerning his/her treatment.
- Have all records and communications regarding medical treatment kept confidential.
- Expect the hospital, within the limits of its capabilities, to respond to a request for services.
- Obtain information regarding the relationship of the hospital to any other health care institutions.
- Be advised if the hospital proposes human experimentation which affects his/her care.
- Reasonable continuity of care.
- An explanation of the bill, regardless of payment source.
- Know what hospital rules and regulations apply to patient contact.

You also have a right to Emergency Room (ER) care. A hospital cannot turn you away if you're having a medical emergency—no matter what insurance coverage you have, or even if you're uninsured. A 1986 federal law, the Emergency Medical Treatment and Labor Act, prohibits hospitals from refusing to examine and stabilize patients in the Emergency Room, even if they cannot pay. In 1998, the federal government ruled that hospitals must ensure immediate care whether or not your HMO or health insurance company approves the treatment—even if the plan says it requires permission before treatment.

"Despite the terms of any managed care agreements . . . federal law requires that stabilizing medical treatment be provided in an emergency," said the Inspector General of the U.S. Department of Health and Human Services. No managed-care contract "can excuse a hospital from providing needed emergency medical screening and stabilizing care."

Additionally, many states have a "prudent layperson" standard that says your health plan must pay for your ER visit if a prudent layperson would have felt the need to seek emergency treatment.

We do recommend that you or an advocate call your health plan as soon as possible, before or after going to the hospital for emergency treatment. Because of a few major lawsuit verdicts against them, health plans are less likely to turn down legitimate ER requests.

From one prudent layperson to another, go out and get the care you need. Don't let health plan regulations frighten you to death.

5.

What to Do When You Have Problems

Three Words:
Document, Complain, and Appeal

WE WANT TO BELIEVE THAT IF WE GET SICK, GREAT MEDICAL care will be there waiting for us. That is often true—but not always.

Most health care organizations are run as businesses, by businesses. They focus on their bottom line, just as you do in your own business and personal finances. By the same token, you are the consumer of health care, and if you (and your employer) have paid for services, then you deserve them. You should not have to beg or plead.

If you're dissatisfied with the services you are receiving, or if you're being denied services you need, then you have every right and reason to complain. We strongly suggest that you document everything. Put your complaints in writing and send them to a specific person by certified mail with a return receipt requested. Maintain a log of all communications, with notations about when you called and to whom you spoke. Keep the log, letters, and other paperwork in one easily accessible place. We suggest starting a "health file," which we'll discuss later in this chapter.

Whenever a health care company denies you anything, ask that they put it in writing. Then, if they don't reply, you can note that they refused to officially respond. If they do send a letter, it might contain something in the wording that you can use to your benefit.

One claims assistance professional told us that she prefers writing letters to making telephone calls. She says, "I do a fair amount of letter writing because if you call, you spend a lot of time on hold. Also, you often don't get the same person twice, and the second person may not agree with what the first person told you. So I send a letter with a return receipt requested. I especially do that with Medicare, because it's such a huge bureaucracy."

All of this is a hassle, we know—and the last thing you want to think about when battling illness. But having this documentation can mean the difference between receiving good services and not getting what you need.

Complain to the health care company first. Be calm, and give details. Ask for a written response within 30 days. If you don't hear back, write or call again. Follow whatever complaint procedure the company has in place. Look in your member handbook for details, or discuss the process with the company's customer service or your employer's benefits department.

Always write down the name of the person you speak to at the health plan. Also, always ask that person for the name of a supervisor. Ask for the spelling of all names. That puts customer service on notice that you're a serious customer, while at the same time ensuring that you have the name of someone to contact the next time you call. Save any phone bills that list long-distance calls to the company.

If you're denied a medical service, find out if there is an "external review" process where your case is examined by an outsider with no financial connection to the plan. These reviews are increasingly common, and more than 30 states now mandate them in certain situations. You are more likely to get a fair shake from an unbiased expert than from a representative of a health plan where the focus is on saving money.

All of this may help, and it may not. A reporter documented cases where health plans simply refused to act on complaints in a timely manner, knowing that most people would give up. Another writer found that many insurance companies deny payments on claims as long as they think they can get away with it, so that they can keep the money earning interest in their bank accounts!

Don't give up. You have many more options. If you have health coverage through an employer, talk to contacts in your employee benefits department, and have them use their pull with the health care company. You can contact city and state regulators, your local elected officials, and the news media, all of whom are now very sensitive to cases where people are denied treatment by health plans.

When you have problems, your documentation will really pay off. You may be able to get an advocate on your side simply by sending over copies of your letters and phone logs.

- If you're not getting the medical care you need, complain to your State Department of Health.
- If you're not getting the benefits you deserve, complain to your State Insurance Department.
- If you believe that your health plan has broken laws or regulations, complain to your State Attorney General. Many cities and states also have a Public Advocate or Consumer Commissioner who can investigate health care problems.
- If you purchased health coverage through an insurance agent or broker, call them up and ask for help or at least advice on the best strategies to pursue.
- If you're in a self-funded health plan, call the Pension and Welfare Benefit Administration (PWBA) of the U.S. Department of Labor.
- In extreme cases, consult a lawyer to learn about your legal recourse. Even in cases that aren't extreme, it could be helpful to have a lawyer send a letter stating your side of

the story. Your health care company might become much more receptive when it sees a letter on legal stationery.

When should you consult a lawyer? According to William Shernoff, a lawyer who has successfully represented health consumers, "When you reach a point where your claim or request for treatment is denied, and after you've tried to get a letter from your doctor, then consult a lawyer. Let's say that someone has cancer and needs a bone marrow transplant, and they go through all these hoops and get a letter that says, 'sorry, we're not going to give it to you because it's experimental and investigational.' Then you need to get a lawyer quick to help you get the treatment, or to give you advice about getting the treatment and then seeking reimbursement later."

To find a lawyer, contact bar associations or local not-for-profit organizations that may have dealt with similar situations. Look for a lawyer who has experience in taking on health care companies. Shernoff warns, "If you have a group medical plan, most lawyers will not take the case, because you can't get anywhere in court. Go to your family lawyer to find out who specializes in this area. It's not a big niche."

In his book *Fight Back & Win: How to Get Your HMO and Health Insurance to Pay Up*, Shernoff suggests that in every letter you send to your health plan, you include the sentence: "This appeal relates only to the denial of the benefits in question, but does not constitute, and shall in no way be deemed, an admission that I am limited in my right to pursue a 'bad faith' remedy in state court." He also notes that 10% of all insurance claims are unjustly denied, but that fewer than 1% of people even ask questions when their claims are refused.

In terms of elected representatives, you can contact your city council member, state senator or assembly member, and U.S. representative or senator. For names and telephone numbers of your elected officials, check your local telephone book or call your local office of the League of Women Voters.

The news media are eager to cover human interest stories about health care. Do you remember hearing about the applause that erupted in many movie theaters during Helen Hunt's anti-HMO speech in *As Good As It Gets?* Frustration with the health care bureaucracy is a topical issue. Before you contact the media, though, make sure that you would feel comfortable discussing your medical condition in public.

Don't be afraid to call on any of these resources. It's unfortunate that people need to resort to this. But it's not your fault if health care companies refuse to provide the services they promised. You deserve to get what you paid for.

Health care bureaucracies can be defeated. As Dr. Bruce Barron writes in his book *Outsmarting Managed Care*, "I have lost count of the number of times I had to do battle with managed care organizations over patient care issues that ranged from the minute to the monumental. The striking thing about each and every one is that, in every instance, the managed care organization caved."

Why Customer Service Is So Bad— And How You Can Get Better Service

Health care is the largest service industry in this country—yet it has just about the worst customer service. One health consumer told us, "I think these customer service people are the ones who couldn't get jobs at McDonalds."

Considering how important health care is for most people, why do health care companies have such terrible customer service?

To a large extent, it's because the people who are directly paying health care bills—employers and government agencies—are not the people receiving the care and having problems with the service. So health care companies put little money or training into their customer service departments.

The bottom line is that your phone call to the Customer Service Department might just be an initial step in getting the service you need. Many of the customer service reps are poorly trained and don't have the power to solve your problems. Sometimes they are downright unhelpful.

One employee benefits person told us about a recent experience: "Four of our policyholders were kept on hold anywhere from 25 to 50 minutes each time they tried to call X Insurance Company—and they tried more than once. Finally, fed up, they called me as their benefits administrator. I, in turn, called a contact of mine in marketing at the company. She gave me the scoop. Seems that X Insurance Company was monitoring their customer service lines and showed documentation that all calls were answered in under two minutes. Yes, the phone was picked up within two minutes, but then the customer was placed on hold for up to 50 minutes. Based on this documentation, they fired 37 customer service representatives. But the situation only got worse now that they fired all these people."

If you call a catalog firm or a travel company, you will probably speak to a cheerful and knowledgeable representative who has been trained to deal with consumers. The customer rep is ready to help you and has the ability to make decisions. However, if you call a health care company, you will likely get stuck on hold and then talk to a surly customer service person who doesn't seem to know what she's talking about.

Expert Ellen Severoni notes, "Quite often the people in customer service are not qualified to answer the complex questions that arise. These are often the least skilled workers in the health plan. In every other service industry, there is power in customer service. Not in health care. People in customer service do not have the power to correct things."

She contrasts this with her veterinarian: "You'd be amazed at the level of service from veterinarians—because people pay out of pocket. We get postcards from our vet all the time telling us about shots and all sorts of things!"

Severoni's group, California Health Decisions, has developed a "best practices" system for customer service. It recommends that when a customer calls a health care company with a problem, the customer service rep should take responsibility for solving it and should stay on top of the problem until it is corrected. If the problem originates from elsewhere (a doctor's office or a lab or another health care practice), the customer service rep should put all of the involved parties on a conference call, including the consumer. The problem should not be "handed off" until someone else has taken responsibility for solving it and informed the consumer.

Wouldn't it be great if all health care customer service representatives did this? You should judge your health plan's services against these "best practices" guidelines and let their reps know when they're falling down on the job. Some customer service reps are truly helpful, but unfortunately they seem to be the exception.

We encourage health care companies to put more emphasis on customer service, but we're realistic enough to know that this won't happen soon. So we encourage you to shift your attitude: Rather than expecting customer service reps to help you and then being frustrated that they don't, understand that they probably won't help you and get ready to go over their heads as soon as possible.

Here's a good tactic. If you're not getting help from the customer service rep, ask for the name and title of the head of the customer service department, and then ask to speak to that person right away. If you can't get through, tell the rep that if you don't hear back from that person by the end of the workday, you will report the company to the Insurance Department. Document everything.

Be aggressive. When you make phone calls or write letters, picture the part of your life where you feel most empowered—whether that's running a marathon, getting a big account, or elbowing people out of the way at a department store sale. With this shift in attitude, you're more likely to get good customer service in a bad-service environment.

Here's a sample letter that you can use to correspond with customer service. After you have sent a letter to a specific person by certified mail with return receipt requested, call a few days later to make sure it arrived on that person's desk. To save yourself time, be prepared to fax another copy of your letter when you call, in case the first one was misplaced. Then wait a week or two and make a second follow-up call to that person to find out the status of your complaint. This time press for action. Find out how quickly the matter can be resolved. You can also ask if there's someone else you could call in customer service to help move things along. If after taking all this action you're still not making progress, it's time to get help elsewhere.

Keep that little green return-receipt slip by the phone so that if anyone claims they never received your letter, you can prove them wrong immediately.

Sample Letter: Complaint about Quality of Care

[Date]
[Your Medical Group or Health Plan]
Customer Service Department
[address]
RE: Grievance of **[your name]**
Subscriber #**[your number]**

Dear Customer Service Department:
    I am writing to express my dissatisfaction with services I received from **[name of provider]** on **[date]**.
    I am unhappy with the services provided by **[name of provider]** for the following reasons: {**Describe the problem you experienced, how it impacted your health, and why you feel the problem should not have occurred or what should have been done differently; include any relevant date(s) and**

any names of people involved, and any actions you have already undertaken attempting to resolve the problem.}

I would appreciate it if you would investigate this matter and take appropriate action to prevent the problem from happening again. You may contact me at [telephone number] if you would like any additional information. Please notify me in writing of the results of your investigation.

Sincerely,
[Your name]
cc: {Possible individuals and/or groups to whom you can consider sending copies of your letter:}
[Health Plan Medical Director]
[Medical Group Medical Director]
[State disciplinary or licensing board]
[Your doctor]
[Party you are complaining about]
[Your employer or insurance broker]
[State regulatory agency]
Attachment(s): {list and attach any written documentation that supports your complaint}

© 1999 Center for Health Care Rights, Los Angeles. Reprinted with permission.

Find Allies in the Health System

The health care system can be confusing, frustrating, and intimidating. Fortunately help is out there for you.

Whenever possible, try to find a real live human being with whom you can make a personal connection. Just as it's important to have a good relationship with your doctor, you want to find an advocate who will know you as an individual and be able to fight for your personal needs. The health care system is often a cold place for an individual battling illness, so look for a warm person who can guide you through it.

A health ally can also provide "professional" backup when you have problems. If you have been denied a service by your health plan, for instance, your health ally might be able to get the decision reversed because of her inside knowledge of medical terminology, insurance forms, or official procedures.

Such a person is more likely to stay on your side if you treat her with respect, thank her for her efforts, stay calm, and follow through on what you say. For example, if an ally is helping you in a conflict with a health plan, and you tell her that you will forward a letter you received rejecting a treatment, then fax or mail the letter that same day. Make it easy for people to help you. A patient advocate told us, "There was one customer service rep I've dealt with a lot over the years, and she's been very helpful to the people I work with. At one point I could tell that there was a strain, and we were both feeling a little tired of each other. So that Christmas I sent her a box of candy, and I got a really nice card back from her."

Julie joined a new health plan not long ago and was bewildered by the paperwork. She couldn't get good answers from customer service until she came across one representative she liked. So she wrote down that woman's name and telephone number at the customer service center in North Dakota. Now, whenever Julie has a problem, she calls that representative, whom she considers "my friend in North Dakota."

Almost anyone can become a Health Ally. Here are some people who may be able to help:

- **Your doctor.** Some doctors view being a patient advocate as part of their job. They will battle the health plan on your behalf. Doctors are usually the best advocates because they know the system inside out and their opinions carry legitimacy. If you have such a doctor, treasure her! But understand that some doctors will be reluctant to take on managed-care corporations or insurance companies because they depend on these businesses for much of their income.

- **Your doctor's staff.** The nurses and receptionists in your doctor's office have dealt with situations similar to yours in the past, and can offer inside advice about what works best. Ask if they can intercede on your behalf. Also find out if they have an "inside contact" at the insurance or managed care company—a real person with a telephone number.

- **Customer service.** Although customer service in health care is famously bad, there are some well-meaning people working there, like Julie's friend in North Dakota. If you find one representative who you can call again, you're likely to get better results.

- **Patient representatives.** Many hospitals and even some health plans have patient representatives (or "ombudsmen") whose job it is to help consumers. Take full advantage of them.

- **Community organizations.** Many of your local not-for-profit community service organizations have highly dedicated staff members experienced in helping people get services.

- **Employers.** Your employer can be an effective advocate, especially if you have a good contact in the benefits department.

- **Employee Assistance Programs (EAPs).** If your employer offers an EAP, use the service when you need help getting the right health care.

- **Unions.** Some unions provide support services for people facing health crises.

- **Government agencies.** We have found the employees of state health and insurance departments to be quite helpful. You can turn to them even before you have a major problem so that you understand your consumer protections and legal rights in advance of contacting a health care company.

- **Local elected officials.** Every elected official from a city council member to your U.S. Senator has staff members ready to help constituents with problems. Health care is consistently ranked as a major political issue, so politicians are very sensitive to their constituents' needs. We can assure you that your health plan will take notice if a Senator's office calls.

Create a Circle of Patient Advocates

One of the most dramatic developments during the AIDS epidemic was the way in which groups of ill individuals and their friends banded together to fight for good care. In the early days of the epidemic, when little was known about the disease, people with AIDS faced enormous stigma and had very few treatment options. Rather than give up and descend into hopelessness, people with AIDS and their supporters created remarkable networks of support groups, service organizations, and formal assistance programs. They also created informal circles of caring. Through these networks, people supported each other, learned very rapidly about treatment advances, heard about the best doctors and hospitals, and found ways to face the most difficult situations.

Paul saw more than once that when a person with AIDS was in the hospital, that person's entire support group would come to visit and offer encouragement. Talk about having good patient advocates! These visitors were the best advocates because they already knew so much about illness themselves.

The support systems created by people with AIDS, and later by women with breast cancer and men with prostate cancer, are models that everyone can use. Not all of us can be doctors or nurses, but anyone can be a patient advocate. We are all patients at some point and we know what that entails, so we are all qualified to be advocates.

The only thing worse than dealing with a medical crisis is

dealing with it alone. There's no need to go through it alone. If you aren't getting support from your relatives and friends, there are other places to turn. Sometimes loved ones are unable to provide support because of their own fears, and you need to look elsewhere. Even the most geographically and emotionally isolated people can find support groups and services. And now with the Internet, that support can come from all over the world.

A remarkable example of a circle of patient advocates is found in the story of Jeanne Sather, a woman with two young sons who underwent treatment for breast cancer. She says, "We kept a list by the phone, and whenever anyone asked if they could do anything, we put their name and phone number on the list. Then we wrote down a separate list of things to be done. One friend took the responsibility of managing that list—of things to be done—and giving assignments to the people from the other list. Another person managed meals. Dinner just showed up at 5 P.M. every day; quite often I didn't even know where it came from. Another person made phone calls to my friends to let them know how I was doing—so I didn't have to make thirty different calls.

"My best recommendation in terms of survival strategies is to make a list and have someone else manage it. Going into something like this, you don't know how much help you'll need." Jeanne is now in remission, and she and her sons recently took a trip to Hawaii to celebrate.

Creating a circle of patient advocates could be the best gift you ever give to a loved one—or to yourself.

Start Your "Health File"

Paperwork often defeats the best health care consumers. People can be informed and assertive while dealing with other people—but then they drown in forms, bills, manuals, brochures, letters, and other documents. So they give up in frustration.

We recommend that you once again take a simple step now to save yourself many headaches down the line. Start a Health File. Begin to build up your own medical record along with all of the paperwork you will need someday. Get an accordion file, or a three-ring binder, or a folder with colored tabs—whatever you use to store papers. Write "My Health File" on the front of it. Then mark off these sections:

- Medical Record
- Health Plan Information (including plan manual and any correspondence you receive from the plan)
- Doctor Information
- Other Doctors/Specialists
- Hospital Information
- Bills
- Nutrition
- Weight Control
- Fitness

You might want to create sections for other members of your family. Or you could start a new Health File for each of them. Add sections for particular conditions, medications, diets, immunizations, etc. "Most people have no idea of their vaccine status for things like tetanus," a doctor told us. Customize and personalize the Health File to meet your needs.

Now put in all the health-related material you have lying around your home. And as paperwork comes in over the months and years, add it to the appropriate section.

Pretty soon you'll have your entire "health portfolio" within easy reach. Then, when you get a bill you don't understand, or a letter that asks you for old papers, all you have to do is look in the file. If you ever need to appeal a health plan decision, you'll have a stack of background papers to send along with your appeal letter—increasing your chances of winning.

Most importantly, you will begin to build your own medical record, along with the records of people you care for (including children and aging parents). We recommend that you periodically order copies of your medical records from your doctors. You have a legal right to obtain, copy, and keep your own records. There may be a fee for photocopying papers and test results or duplicating x-rays, but it's well worth the cost. Considering the sorry state of information-keeping in the health care field, you will probably do a better job of maintaining your medical file than anyone else. In the future, you'll be more likely to win appeals based on "medical necessity" if you can send copies of your medical records along with the appeal letter. Don't let anyone contest your right to get all of your medical records—patient access is guaranteed by law.

If a doctor ever said that he couldn't do anything for you until he received your medical records from another office, wouldn't it be good to say, "Oh, I brought a copy of my file along. I have it right here!" And if you ever needed to rush a loved one to the Emergency Room, wouldn't it be great to take his whole health history with you, rather than waiting for a clerk in the ER to try to track down far-flung files in the middle of the night?

Are Your Medical Records Private?

We have little medical privacy. Our medical records are often obtained by employers, insurance companies, and even private detectives. This is yet another area where consumers "assume" that laws and regulators protect them. For the most part, it's not true.

There's only one way to keep visits to doctors, mental health professionals, and hospitals completely private—but it's extreme. If you absolutely do not want anyone to know, then use a fake name and pay for everything in cash. That's what actor Brad Davis did when he received treatment for AIDS. He believed that if people knew he had AIDS, he would never get another acting job. Because of his secrecy, the press didn't learn about his condition until he died.

A less drastic approach is to carefully monitor your medical records. Once a year, request your file from medical providers, and make sure that all of the entries are accurate. If you find anything wrong, request in writing that the provider remove it. Also request in writing that providers give out as little information as possible from your medical record. For instance, if you have an insurance claim, your provider should only send the relevant pages from your file rather than sending the entire file. And don't sign a "blanket waiver" giving anyone complete access to your medical records. You can and should edit such a release form before signing it.

Talk to your doctor about sensitive information that you wouldn't want a prospective employer to see, like drug use or sexually transmitted diseases. If you have a good relationship with your doctor, you can ask her to not make notes about these issues in your medical record. Remember that you will need to inform other doctors in the future about the same issues.

If you're seeing a psychiatrist or mental health professional, you may want to have the same discussions about your record. Some managed care companies have demanded copies of records in order to reimburse therapists, leaving your most sensitive information open to accidental disclosure. A recent survey found that more than one-third of therapists had a patient who paid out of pocket specifically because of fear of disclosure.

How did we get to the point that people are afraid of their medical records being leaked? Hippocrates counseled doctors to keep their patients' secrets "sacred," and medical privacy has always been an important part of health care. But people don't feel that their medical records will be kept private. According to a national poll by Princeton Survey Research Associates, only 35% of us feel that our health plan will keep information confidential "all or most of the time." Only 33%

feel that our records will be protected in government programs like Medicare.

They're right to be concerned. No federal law prevents the selling or trading of your medical records. State laws are a patchwork of legislation, much of it ineffectual. In a Louis Harris poll of health care professionals, 34% said medical records were given to unauthorized people somewhat often. If companies want to get your medical records, they probably can. And some businesses do—ranging from insurance companies and pharmacy benefit managers (PBMs) to employers and prospective employers. In fact, a study in the *Employment Rights and Employment Policy Journal* found that 35% of large employers consider medical information when making employment decisions.

Even more chilling, private investigators have reported that they can obtain medical records by paying off workers at insurance companies and doctor's offices. These actions are illegal but the potential penalties aren't strong enough to frighten dishonest health care workers.

Our personal experience confirms that medical privacy is sorely lacking. Julie saw numerous medical file mix-ups while being treated for cancer. Paul recently called the office of a doctor he hadn't seen in several years to ask for a copy of his old medical record. He was shocked when a receptionist said, "Sure!" without requesting identification or authentication.

If you have recently applied for health insurance, there may be a file on you at the MIB. No, that's not the Men In Black, but the Medical Information Bureau. This company was founded in 1902 by a group of doctors who worked at insurance companies. It has been collecting information ever since, and claims to have reports for about 15% of health insurance applicants. You can find out if the MIB has a file on you by calling (617) 426-3660 or going to www.mib.com.

The MIB will do a search for $8.50. You can have the charge waived if you meet any of the following conditions:

(1) You were recently turned down for life, health, or disability insurance, or were charged an extra premium, and MIB was the information source; (2) You are unemployed and plan to seek employment in the next 60 days; (3) You are on welfare; (4) Your MIB record is inaccurate due to fraud. If you find errors in your file, you can ask to have them corrected. MIB claims to fix errors within 30 days of being notified.

If you're adamant that no one learn about your medical condition, then use an assumed name and pay cash. Otherwise, protect yourself as much as possible by discussing the issue with your doctor, keeping your own medical file, examining your providers' records, and understanding that your privacy is limited.

"This Bill Came a Year Late from a Doctor I Never Heard of for a Procedure I Never Had," or Why Bills Don't Make Sense, and What You Can Do about It

It would be funny if it weren't so serious. Health care billing is notoriously slow, incomplete, and difficult to understand—and often involves large amounts of money!

We have never been able to get a good explanation as to why health care billing is so bad, other than the generally poor state of information systems and computer technology in the medical sector combined with the previously discussed bad customer service. Ironically, billing is an area where patients in HMOs often fare better than those in Fee-for-Service, because tightly controlled managed care plans eliminate much of the paperwork for in-network visits.

There are steps you can take to protect yourself. First, check all bills carefully. Hospital bills are especially known to be filled with errors. Investigative writer Martin L. Gross notes, "Stories of fifteen dollars for an aspirin are quite true, mainly because the hospital bill really is a piece of fiction."

You should contest in writing any charge you disagree with or don't understand. Don't pay for the bill until you have a clear response. Health care companies may not put a diagnosis on the bill, for privacy reasons, but you should still be able to understand what the charges are for.

One health expert told us confidentially that he knows of hospitals which use "default billing," where they automatically add fees and taxes that may not apply to you. Review any extra fees that look "automatic" very carefully. If you're going to be responsible for a major part of a large bill, then you might want to hire a professional to review the bill for you. This person could be a lawyer or an accountant, or a claims assistance professional, which is described below. Although you'll be charged for a professional's time, you could save much more money than you pay in fees. Reduced charges could also help you avoid reaching your lifetime cap on medical expenses.

Many people have told us how frustrated they feel when they get a bill in the mail one year—or more—after they received the medical service. Unfortunately, there aren't time limits on medical bills, so you can get bills a year or two later. These bills usually come from laboratories, or specialists, or ambulances—services that are the "second or third tier" away from the patient. Anesthesiologists are also big offenders here. Some of these people seem to not be able to get their paperwork done in a timely fashion. To be fair to them, though, some have to wait a long time to get needed paperwork from the doctors or hospitals. So the bad news is that you usually do still have to pay the bill. The good news is that your insurance should still reimburse you.

If the bill is just inaccurate, then document, complain, and appeal. If they can wait a year and a half to bill you, they can wait a few months for the bill to be appealed.

Paul once started getting bills from a medical institution he had not visited in more than two years, for unidentified services on a date long after he had seen a doctor there. He just ignored the first bill, figuring it was so obviously wrong that the billing department would realize its mistake. When a statement referring to that bill came a month later, he responded with a letter saying that the bill was not valid. Then the statements started coming every month. Every month, Paul would write "NOT VALID—SEE MY PREVIOUS LETTER" on the statement and then send it back in the preaddressed envelope. And the statements kept coming. At one point, he was tempted to just pay the bill, because it was a comparatively small amount. But he felt offended by the idea of paying for a service he hadn't received. So he kept sending the statements back to the billing office. Eventually they stopped coming. What happened? Who knows—but he never paid a dime, other than the cost of a few stamps.

"Many bills are incomprehensible," says Susan Dressler, CCAP, president of the Alliance of Claims Assistance Professionals. This trade organization is for professionals who represent individuals regarding billing disputes and payment problems with health care companies. "You would think someone would be able to design a standard bill—but I've never seen one," Dressler comments. "There are a lot of elements that get dropped or forgotten, and other pieces that we have to put together."

If you don't understand a bill, ask for an itemized bill. You don't have to accept whatever the company sends you first. Usually when you ask for an itemized bill, you will receive an "HCFA 1500," which is the closest thing to a standard form that exists.

In fact, it's always best to ask for an itemized bill, even for a doctor's visit. You want to see exactly what you're being charged for. It's not uncommon to be charged for expensive tests that you never had. Neither you nor your insurer should have to pay for such mistakes.

Most billing problems are the result of human error. At times, fraud is involved. If you suspect that you're the victim of fraud, respond aggressively. Even if a third party is paying the bill, we all pay for health care fraud through higher taxes and insurance premiums. There are also "whistleblower" statutes that mean you can collect a reward or a percentage of money retrieved from perpetrators. The Office of the Inspector General of the Department of Health and Human Services has instituted a formal Fraud Hotline at (800) 447-8477.

If you keep getting bills that are inaccurate and you can't get any answers from the billing department of the health care company, it's time to call in the troops. Go to your state insurance department; for contact information, see the listings in Appendix C. Put everything in writing and ask the department to investigate.

An even better strategy is to start sending the Insurance Department copies of every letter you send your health plan at the same time you send the original letters. That way you create a paper trail, and putting "cc: State Insurance Department" at the bottom of a letter will get the attention of the company.

When you deal with Insurance Department employees, remember that they are government workers who are probably civil servants. Many of these employees feel overworked and underpaid, so you may have to push your situation forward. While you might find some dedicated employees, they don't necessarily have an incentive to provide the best customer service themselves.

This is another place to find a Health Ally. Present a compelling case about how the insurance company is mistreating you, and how you must get the help of the Insurance Department to set things right. However frustrated you feel towards your insurance company or health plan, don't take it out on the people who can help you. Always be reasonable, calm, and courteous. If you sincerely thank them for their help, they will be much more likely to remain on your side.

Find out where your insurance company has its headquarters. If the insurance company has its headquarters in a different state, then you may well need to approach the insurance department in that state. Send copies of your letters to the insurance commissioners in both states. However callous the companies may be, they don't want to needlessly attract the attention of the insurance commissioners.

In plans that are self-insured (where large companies take the "risk" for payments on themselves), you're not covered by state insurance laws but rather by the federal law known as ERISA. Your state insurance commissioner will not be able to help you. Instead, you should contact the Pension and Welfare Benefit Administration (PWBA). It's more difficult to pursue individual cases there, but it's still worth trying.

The health care companies don't make it easy to get answers—or even to get through to a live person to discuss the problems. Dressler, who worked in insurance claims departments for 20 years, notes that "now there is less human intervention with claims than ever before. People are left in the middle of nowhere because of a lack of true human communication. I had someone call me recently and ask if I was a real person. He was so shocked that a real human being answered the phone."

If you don't feel you can defend yourself against inaccurate billing, or if you don't have the time or energy to properly process all of the paperwork and make the phone calls, you can hire a claims professional. Most charge on an hourly basis, with rates ranging from $20 to $60 per hour. Hire someone with an insurance background because the material is very technical and you want someone who knows all the details. For a referral, you can contact the Alliance of Claims Assistance Professionals or the American Health Information Management Association. Both are listed in Appendix A. You can also look into web sites which offer similar services, including www.HealthAllies.com.

After she had become exhausted by dealing with billing problems, cancer survivor Jeanne Sather found a claims professional in the Yellow Pages under Medical Claims. "I did really well on managing my own medical care," Sather says, "but the billing defeated me. There were many errors, and almost always the errors were in their favor. I got one bill for $1,700, with the explanations all in codes. Under the Patient Responsibility line, it said I owed all $1,700! I knew that if I didn't do anything, it would keep coming back to me." By hiring a claims professional, Jeanne figures that she saved many times what she paid in fees.

The woman Jeanne hired is Kelly Calden of Edmonds, Washington. Calden says, "When I start going through someone's piled-up bills, it's like a jigsaw puzzle. So I create my own statements, which is like keeping a journal. When I call insurers for information, I always write down who I talk to and what they say. Sometimes I'll go and buy a big calendar, and write down everything that happens for a client day-by-day. And I try to get my clients as involved as they can be in the process."

She adds, "My service usually pays for itself by getting clients the benefits. I stay on top of it. I'm sure that at a certain point people say, 'I'm going to take care of this before that woman calls me again!' I always remain calm and professional, but I'm very determined."

Calden says that the most important things to remember about billing are: (1) Establish right away what services are covered by your health plan; (2) Don't pay your bills before the insurance company does; (3) Make sure that your doctors have your current insurance information; (4) Carry that information around with you at all times; (5) Don't let bills pile up without doing anything about it; and (6) Never let your health insurance lapse.

That last point is particularly important for anyone dealing with a health crisis. Calden has seen some ill people let bills pile up unopened for months. Sometimes the bill for their health insurance is in that pile, and so coverage gets cancelled.

It's also important to make sure that your insurers and providers know where you are. Calden worked with one older gentleman who went into a nursing home. His mail was not getting forwarded—so he wasn't paying his premiums and very nearly lost his coverage.

Here's a good sample letter to use when you have billing problems:

Sample Letter: Billing Problems

[Date]
[Your Medical Group or Health Plan]
Customer Service Department
[address]
RE: Appeal for **[your name]**
Subscriber #**[your number]**

Dear Customer Service Department:

I am writing to request that **[name of medical group OR health plan]** cover a bill I received for **[service, treatment, OR procedure]**. The service was provided on [date] by [name of provider (**doctor, lab, hospital, other**)] to address **[medical problem]**. The bill I received is for **[dollar amount]** and must be paid by **[date]**. I believe this bill should be covered by my [medical group OR health plan]. I called the [medical group OR health plan] on [date(s)], and I spoke with [name of representative] concerning the bill, but the problem has not yet been resolved.

I believe this bill should be paid by [name of medical group OR health plan] because: {List specific reasons you think the bill should be paid. Possible reasons are listed below. Choose as many reasons to include in your letter as apply to you. The first reason probably should be included in any billing letter.}

- [name of service] is a covered service under my health plan coverage terms;
- a referral for [service, treatment, OR procedure] was provided by my primary care physician;
- [service, treatment, OR procedure] was performed by my primary care physician;
- [service, treatment, OR procedure] was performed by a specialist to whom I was referred by my primary care physician;
- the services were medically necessary;
- there are no coverage exclusions or limitations of [service, treatment, OR procedure], or that apply to my case;
- I have met all of my co-payment or deductible obligations under the health plan's coverage terms;
- I could not get prior authorization before receiving [service, treatment, OR procedure] because my health care problem was an emergency. I did call my [primary care physician, health plan, or medical group] as soon as I could after receiving the [service, treatment, OR procedure], as required by my health plan.

The [medical group OR health plan's] failure to pay the bill violates [federal AND/OR state] law which requires [applicable legal requirement]. {You can refer to the code section under the law that applies. For example, HMOs in California are required to pay for certain services: (See Cal. Health & Safety Code § [code number].)}

Attached is documentation supporting your responsibility for the bill.

Please respond in writing and let me know what actions you will take regarding this request. Thank you for your prompt attention to this matter.

Sincerely,

[Your name]

cc: {Possible individuals and/or groups to whom you can consider sending copies of your letter are:}

[Your primary care physician]

[Billing party]

[Medical group]

[Health plan]

[Your employer or insurance broker]

[State regulatory agency]

Attachments: Copy of bill dated [date]

{Other material and documentation you can consider attaching are:}

Copies of portions of plan member handbook or EOC stating coverage terms, (i.e. specific coverage provisions, and/or definition of medical necessity and list of exclusions and limitations);

Copy of referral;

Copy of letter from doctor;

Medical records;

Medical journal articles supporting medical necessity of care received.

© 1999 Center for Health Care Rights, Los Angeles. Reprinted with permission.

How to Send Mail to Health Care Companies

Why should we tell you how to send mail to your health plan, hospital, or other health care organization? You know how to mail a letter, right?

Unfortunately these organizations sometimes claim that mail never reached them—so they don't have to act on requests or complaints. The post office loses very little mail, in our experience. So these companies are either losing mail internally, or receiving mail but then lying about it.

Protect yourself by always sending letters via certified mail, and get a return receipt. If you're willing to spend more, use an express mail service. Keep all of your receipts in an easy-to-find file. Send the letter to a specific person ("Mary Black, Customer Service Manager, X Insurance") rather than just a department ("X Customer Service Department"). Call a few days after the letter should have arrived to confirm that it was received by that person.

We know this is a hassle. But as with many things in health care, spending a little time now can save you a lot of time and aggravation in the future. Quite often there's a "ticking clock" with decisions or appeals required within a certain time frame. Don't let health plans and hospitals stop the "ticking clock" by claiming they never heard from you.

When we wrote our New York consumer health guidebook, we sent a questionnaire to nearly every health plan and hospital in the New York area. Most did not respond. So we called to follow up. Many times the response we got back was "We never received it." So we would pull out our little green return-receipt slip and say, "Yes, you did receive it, and it was signed for on October 29 by so and so." We'll never forget that one PR person at a New York hospital told us, very haughtily, "Just because someone signed for it in the mailroom doesn't mean it ever got to my desk."

When we told a doctor friend that many offices were claiming to have never received our letters, he laughed and said, "Oh yeah, I've used that trick, too." We're not sure which is worse—that people in health care lie about receiving documents, or that a great deal of correspondence may actually get lost in medical facilities.

Even after relentless follow-up calls, only half of the health plans and hospitals would send us any information. We are trying to change the attitude among health care companies that they "own" information and don't have to tell anyone any-thing, but it's a long-term struggle. You will probably encounter that attitude, so protect yourself.

Advice from Your Friends and Neighbors

We recently conducted a survey of how people feel about the health care system and the services they receive. One of the questions we asked was what advice they would give friends about getting the best health care. Here are some of the answers we received:.

> *"Know what you are entitled to under your health plan—read and ask questions. Don't be intimidated by those in power."*

> *"Be very informed about patient's rights, treatment options, and obtaining second opinions."*

> *"Check doctors' medical education, affiliation, years in the field of expertise, and reputation."*

> *"Get a job that has good benefits."*

> *"Contact as many people who are currently using the plan and get as much feedback as possible."*

> *"Start a chart on at least 5 HMOs and study them carefully."*

> *"Ask questions, get it in writing, never assume anything."*

"*Make sure you can pick your own physicians. Make sure you have copies of all your paperwork in dealing with hospitals, doctors, and insurance plans.*"

"*First, check with friends and neighbors to locate a good hospital. Then join an HMO or similar plan that uses that hospital.*"

"*Be prepared to fight for the best care and the most comprehensive care that you need.*"

"*Scrutinize the plans, pay more to get more, and look into options if you should actually be sick—what's covered. Demand good care in hospitals and write letters; praise the good and expose the bad.*"

"*Be persistent!*"

"*Get a long-term care policy now.*"

"*Make sure you know your rights so they won't send you out of the hospital too soon.*"

"*Be sure to audit all charges and dispute any cost which is unreasonable.*"

"*Select a plan which permits you to use the doctors of your choice, and which covers alternative treatments.*"

"*When needed, go to a major teaching hospital.*"

"*Don't be intimidated by the hospital's billing office.*"

"If you are denied reimbursement on a bill, argue; I found 99% of the time my bills were turned down it was either due to a mistake, or the need to reasonably discuss [it]."

"Ask how emergency situations are handled, because people are generally healthy and get sick unexpectedly."

"Get opinions from nurses who really know."

"Complain in writing [by] certified mail [with] return receipts to verify complaints and get results."

"Keep every bill and receipt."

"Get a plan that offers flexibility—it is nice to know you can go to an out-of-network doctor if you have a life-threatening condition."

"Be prepared for a lot of correspondence and a lot of paperwork."

"If on Medicare, take that plus a good supplemental policy."

"Photocopy everything, and do not be pushed around by anybody."

"Move to Canada." [Note: This was a popular response.]

"Read and understand your member handbook. If benefits are denied, appeal the decision; there's a good chance you'll win."

*"Shop around. Do not just go with the least expensive;
be sure the plan will cover exactly what you need."*

*"I would suggest that if they could afford it that they
should apply for a Point Of Service or traditional
indemnity plan and avoid any plan where choice of
doctors is restricted."*

*"Be careful, be informed, be your own advocate or
have someone else do it for you. Remember
you're a consumer."*

*"Do not be intimidated by doctors and always ask
questions if you do not understand what they
are telling you."*

"Find out the ratings of the HMOs."

*"Find a local organization that can help sort out
details when necessary."*

*"Are you married? Think of your lifestyle. Study
[plans] well. Compare the pros and cons
on a chart."*

*"Become informed about your own health and
problems. Be your own best advocate."*

*"Document everything you are told on the phone
(name, time, and date) when calling. If they
think you cannot back up what you say happened,
they will say they have no record of such a thing.
Once you give them documentation, they
do what they were supposed to do
in the first place."*

*"Find your own doctors, or call physician referral
services at hospitals."*

*"Be prepared to 'manage' your health care yourself.
If you join an HMO, you have to be vigilant and
stand up and fight to get what you need at times."*

*"I would tell my friend to choose a medical plan and
hospital like you would your wife. You want the
very best possible."*

"Keep records and complain all the way to the top."

*"Ask for the full plan manual. This is especially true
if you have a family member with special needs."*

*"Keep yourself as healthy as you can. Eat healthy and
exercise. Have a hobby. Have good friends and
laughter so that you can avoid doctors and hospitals."*

6.

How to Save Money and Find Free Services

20 Ways to Save Money on Health Care

HEALTH CARE IS HUGELY EXPENSIVE. ANYONE WHO HAS recently received a medical bill knows that. And the costs you see are only a portion of what you actually spend on health care. Because so much of the payment is indirect and invisible to the consumer (through taxes and monthly premiums at work), most people never realize how much medical spending costs them.

Still, there are effective ways to save money while getting excellent health care. Here are 20 valuable tips:

1. **Be a smart shopper.** Shop around. You have choices in your health care. Even if you can only choose one health plan, you can pick doctors, clinics, pharmacies, hospitals, and other providers. Ask for prices in advance. Be ready to go elsewhere if you don't get straightforward answers.
2. **Join groups and associations.** Many associations, alumni organizations, unions, and other groups offer health care deals that will save you far more than the cost of joining. For instance, if you are eligible, the Veterans of Foreign Wars (VFW) is good at helping veterans navigate the VA system.

3. **Contest bills.** Health care billing is filled with errors. Don't pay a bill until you have a complete explanation of what it's for, and you're certain that all services were provided.

4. **Keep good records.** If you get a bill that doesn't make sense, you will have a paper trail to back up your version of events and to avoid paying overbilled or inaccurate charges.

5. **Negotiate fees.** Yes, you can negotiate fees in many areas of health care, and people do it all the time. "Health care pricing is often bogus," says David Lansky, executive director of the Foundation for Accountability. "It's like airline seats, where the person sitting next to you on an airplane may have paid hundreds of dollars less than you." As we mentioned earlier, you can negotiate with a new employer regarding having it pay your COBRA premiums until you're covered under its health plan. If you want a private room in a hospital, you can negotiate with the hospital about how much extra it will cost you. Hospitals have a lot of empty beds, so you have some bargaining power. If you're going to an out-of-network doctor, find out what the UCR fee is from your health plan and negotiate with the doctor to accept that fee.

6. **Influence your company's benefits.** Get your employee benefits people on your side. Press for more choices, lower costs, and better services.

7. **Keep your health insurance information with you at all times.** Carry the card you get from your plan, or take along a small piece of paper noting the names, policy numbers, and telephone contacts. Put this information in your purse or wallet. Many billing problems arise simply because people don't have their insurance information handy when it's needed.

8. **If you or a family member has a pre-existing condition, be very careful about changing health plans.** Make sure that you understand what will be covered under any new plan

you consider, and what treatment may be "excluded" for a set amount of time. Exclusions vary based on the plan, employer, and state. For more information, contact your state insurance department ahead of time.

9. **When you change jobs or insurers, notify your doctors and other providers right away.** Many billing problems arise because paperwork is mailed to the wrong insurance company—and is then sent to you for "full payment" when reimbursement is turned down elsewhere.

10. **If you can't understand your medical bills, hire a claims assistance professional to take care of it for you.** You will likely save more money than you pay in fees.

11. **Before any surgery or procedure, get a second opinion.** Up to 25% of surgical procedures are unnecessary. Even at renowned cancer hospitals, between 1.4% and 8.8% of biopsies are wrongly diagnosed. If a second opinion saves you from going through an unwarranted operation and its attendant costs and medical risks, it's well worth the trouble. Do let your first doctor know that you're getting a second opinion so that your medical records can be forwarded.

12. **Take tax deductions for health expenses.** If you're self-employed, you can deduct a large portion of your health insurance premiums. If you spent a sizeable percentage of your income on medical expenses in one year, you may be able to deduct these expenses. Consult an accountant to find out what deductions are permitted.

13. **Find free services at community organizations.** Affinity groups like the American Legion, church groups, and the Presbyterian Church are doing a lot to promote health care quality. Organizations such as the American Cancer Society, the National Breast Cancer Coalition, and the Arthritis Foundation have become very good at providing consumer service. Use the not-for-profit community health organizations in your local area. Also, attend community health fairs, which offer free blood pressure readings and

other free or low-cost screening tests. There are thousands of health-related not-for-profit organizations in this country, and many are visible at these fairs.

14. **Use government programs.** A growing percentage of American families are eligible for these programs. That's not surprising, because nearly half of all health care spending in the U.S. comes from government. Some people have told us that there's a stigma about being in a government health program like Medicaid (for people with low incomes), CHIP (Child Health Insurance Program), and ADAP (prescription drug assistance program). It's time to get beyond that. Almost everyone over 65 is on Medicare, which is one of the most popular of all government programs. Medicaid pays bills for two-thirds of the elderly in nursing homes. You have been paying taxes to support these health programs for years, so don't hesitate to enroll when you're eligible. Check with local government agencies; you may be surprised by the number of programs for which your family is eligible. CHIP is a great program for kids—and no child should go without health insurance. Call (877) KIDS-NOW for information about CHIP.

15. **Go to government-supported medical clinics.** Quality varies widely at these clinics, from uneven to surprisingly good. Most operate on a sliding scale basis that is affordable to almost everyone. For information, contact your state or city health department.

16. **If you have no money for health care, contact your local Medical Society to ask about free services.** A medical society is an association of doctors. Most states and larger cities have their own medical societies. Call the office in your area and ask if they have a referral service or program for people who can't afford medical care.

17. **Look into clinical trials.** For the testing of some new therapies, the patient's expenses are paid. For more information, contact the National Institutes of Health Clinical

Center's Patient Recruitment and Referral Line at (800) 411-1222 or www.cc.nih.gov. You can also check www.clinicaltrials.gov. Before enrolling in a clinical trial, read all of the forms carefully and make sure that you understand if any risks are involved.

18. **If you need expensive medical care and your health plan won't pay, you can contact the national Medical Care Ombudsman Program at (888) 313-6267 or www.mcman.com.** It may be able to work out a deal with your health plan. The service is free to those who cannot afford to pay. Or contact the Center for Patient Advocacy at (800) 846-7444 or www.patientadvocacy.org. You can also call your local bar association and community based organizations to request free legal assistance.

19. **If you were in a hospital and can't afford to pay the bill, ask the hospital about its obligation to provide free services.** The hospital may have obligations under the Hill-Burton Free Care program, a federal government program for low-income persons. For more information, call the Hill-Burton Hospital Free Care Line at (800) 638–0742. Ask the hospital about further obligations under state and local laws. Additionally, some hospitals have funds specifically set aside to pay the bills of people who cannot afford to do so themselves.

20. **Maintain a healthy lifestyle.** Avoid visits to doctors and hospitals by practicing basic health habits. Exercise regularly, eat a balanced and nutritious diet that includes a lot of fruits and vegetables, get enough sleep, don't smoke cigarettes, and limit alcohol consumption. Learn about good health and fitness, and educate yourself about your own medical conditions by reading books and articles and by surfing the Internet.

15 Ways to Save Money on Prescription Drugs

One of the biggest issues in health care today is the high cost of prescription drugs. Out of pocket spending on prescription drugs is increasing 8% a year—well ahead of the inflation rate. Here are 15 things you can do to save money:

1. **Compare prices at local pharmacies.** Prices can vary a great deal within the same town or city.
2. **Shop by mail order or online for better bargains.** If you shop online, go to well-known Internet pharmacies like drugstore.com, cvs.com, walgreens.com, and PlanetRx.com. Be wary of smaller Internet companies you've never heard of, and don't order from pharmacies based outside the country. Take shipping charges into account, because they can add a lot to the final bill.
3. **If a doctor suggests a prescription for a new drug, ask how much it costs** and whether there are less expensive alternatives. Make sure that your doctor understands that you need to save money.
4. **Ask your doctor if you can get a prescription for higher-dose pills and cut them in half.** Tablets with twice the potency often cost only 25% to 50% more. You can use an inexpensive "pill cutter" available for purchase at some pharmacies.
5. **When getting a new prescription filled, consider asking the pharmacist for half the amount specified.** That way if you can't tolerate the drug, you're out less money. You can also ask your doctor if she has free medical samples, so that you can test the drug before filling the prescription.
6. **Use the AARP Pharmacy Service,** which offers good prices on brand-name drugs, generics, and over-the-counter items. You don't have to be a member of AARP or over a

specific age. The service accepts most prescription insurance plans, and has a low flat-rate shipping charge. Call (800) 456-2277 or go to www.rpspharmacy.com.

7. **If you live near the border, think about taking a trip to Canada or Mexico to buy pharmaceutical drugs in bulk.** Drugs cost less in other countries because of different laws and regulations.

8. **Ask your health plan to send you its formulary (list of approved drugs).** If it won't do so, ask where you can examine the list or find out if specific medications are on the list. Make sure that your prescription drugs are on the formulary. If they aren't, you may have to pay all or most of the cost of your prescriptions. Can you substitute a medication that's on the formulary? Discuss the possibilities with your doctor. Can you change to another health plan with a better formulary? If changing will save you hundreds of dollars a year, it's an option worth examining. If you're already in a health plan and any prescription is denied, appeal the denial immediately.

9. **Inquire about replacing generic drugs for brand names.** Generics cost much less. Discuss this with your doctor and/or pharmacist.

10. **Ask your doctor and pharmacist if there are over-the-counter drugs that would work as well for your condition.** Some medications that were formerly prescription-only are now available over-the-counter and are much less expensive. Weigh what you would spend for the over-the-counter drug against your co-payment for the prescription medication.

11. **If you're going into a hospital or clinic, you can bring your own medications along.** This includes over-the-counter medications. You may then be spared getting charged $15 per Tylenol tablet. Discuss this with your doctor ahead of time.

12. **Eliminate unnecessary medications.** You may not need to continue all of the drugs you have been on, especially the ones you have been taking for years. Use the "brown paper

bag" test. Visit your doctor and bring your medications in a brown paper bag. Have the doctor see if you need all of them. This exercise could prevent serious problems because some medications are "contraindicated" and should not be taken together. Bring all the vitamins and herbs you take, as well.

13. **Look into drug trials.** With the explosion of pharmaceutical research and testing of new treatments, there are many drugs in the late stages of research. Check with pharmaceutical companies to see if they're testing any drugs for your conditions. Ask your librarian for help in identifying companies. There are drawbacks you should investigate, including potential side effects and the possibility that you may receive a placebo (sugar pill with no active ingredients) as part of a randomized trial.

14. **If you have no money for medications, ask about indigent patient programs.** You can contact pharmaceutical companies directly to ask about their free drug programs. Most people are unaware that pharmaceutical companies give away large amounts of drugs to people who could not otherwise pay. For more information, contact the Pharmaceutical Manufacturer's Association at www.phrma.org/patients.

15. **In many states, seniors and people with life-threatening illnesses qualify for low-cost drug programs.** Benefits and requirements vary, so call your state health department. For contact information, see Appendix C. Also, ask pharmacies about senior discounts.

Free and Low-Cost Services in Your Area

When Julie was diagnosed with cancer, she turned to family and friends—and cancer organizations. "I relied a lot on support systems," she says. "There are support groups, not-for-profit organizations, and many other places you can turn."

Paul worked for not-for-profit AIDS service organizations for five years. He saw literally thousands of people affected by HIV who were helped by excellent services that were provided to them completely free of charge.

Americans are generous people. We may not have the best health care system in the world, but we almost certainly have the best network of not-for-profit health service organizations providing free programs to millions of individuals affected by illnesses and chronic conditions. We strongly urge you to take advantage of the services in your community.

You may not be aware of how many groups exist nearby. The organizations tend to be small and they have little money for advertising, marketing, and promotion. So you may have to go out and find them. That's well worth doing.

These organizations provide a wide array of educational forums, support groups, direct services, financial assistance, insurance counseling, and other programs. Each group is different, so call and ask for information. The employees of these organizations, while often overworked, do sincerely want to help people. They provide a human touch that is missing amidst the coldness of our health care system. Whatever problem you have, they are likely to have seen it before, and can tell you about programs and services which will help.

For every disease and condition, there are organizations. Start by looking in your local phone book. You might also try to speak with a local librarian (great sources of health information!) or do a search on the Internet. Friends and colleagues are good for referrals.

We are strong believers in the value of support groups. From our personal experiences, we know how beneficial support groups can be for people affected by chronic conditions and life-threatening illnesses. Caretakers and loved ones of ill individuals also benefit from help and support, and can now find many services tailored to their specific needs.

Some people are uncomfortable with support groups

because they don't want to share their feelings with strangers. We understand this fear, but want people to know that most support groups are confidential and don't push people to reveal more than they wish.

Support groups can also keep you up on the latest medical developments and give you valuable firsthand feedback about those doctors, hospitals, and other organizations that are doing cutting edge work. Do you want to know the inside scoop on medical services in your town? This is where you'll get it! Receiving current information through the "grapevine" at support groups is a valuable benefit.

We list dozens of not-for-profit organizations in Appendix A. This is actually a short list, because there are tens of thousands of organizations providing free and low-cost health and support services throughout the country. Through the organizations we list, you can learn about many other helpful groups.

Resources for Small Businesses

Small businesses face vexing problems in providing health care to their employees. Most businesses would like to provide health benefits as a way of attracting and keeping skilled workers. But costs can be very high for small businesses, and rate increases are shocking to their bottom line. We have received telephone calls from small business owners who just got notice of double-digit premium increases—sometimes close to triple-digit increases! So the majority of small businesses in this country do not offer their employees health coverage.

The best approach for small businesses is to get "big" by joining with other businesses. The more purchasing power they have, the more likely they are to get better deals from the health plans. Many cities now have purchasing alliances for small businesses. And many small business associations have allied themselves with health plans.

In Northern Ohio, a health insurance program for small

businesses sponsored by the Greater Cleveland Growth Association now reaches over 100,000 employee subscribers within 16,000 small businesses, covering 250,000 people. The program has been around for more than 25 years. As it has grown, the program has been able to negotiate more favorable rates with insurance companies. In addition to offering 18 different health plans to members, it provides dental, vision, disability, and worker's compensation coverage. The program estimates that it saves small businesses $50 million annually. Bigger is better.

Some of the corporations that sell supplies and services to small businesses are getting into health coverage. Our business recently got a solicitation for health insurance from Costco, the large warehouse buying club. We never realized that we could sign up for health insurance at the same place we get huge boxes of toilet paper and cereal. The plan looked like a decent one, too.

For a state-by-state breakdown of information about health insurance for small businesses, go to the web site of Georgetown University's Institute for Health Care Research and Policy at www.georgetown.edu/research/ihcrp/hipaa.

To find out more about Consumer Health Purchasing Groups for small businesses, contact the Institute for Health Policy Solutions in Washington, DC at (202) 789-1491 or www.ihps.org.

And to find out more about group plans in your region, contact all of your local business associations, Chambers of Commerce, and small business support programs.

Free Help for People on Medicare

Medicare is the government-funded health program for people 65 and older and for people with certain disabilities. (It is different from Medicaid, the government-funded health care program for people with low incomes). Medicare is a federal entitlement program funded by payroll taxes.

Medicare is a basic program, focusing on hospitalization, doctor visits, and lab tests. Most other services are excluded, so a number of insurance companies sell "Medigap" plans to fill in the gaps. There are 10 different kinds of Medigap plans, known by the letters Plan A to Plan J.

Many people on Medicare have joined HMOs, which promised greater services while eliminating out-of-pocket costs for items such as prescriptions. In return, HMOs limit choice of providers. Some HMOs have recently abandoned the Medicare market in regions where they were losing money. Many people feel that they were "burned" by Medicare HMOs that made them promises, but later dropped services. Fortunately they were entitled to return to traditional Medicare.

If you're in a Medicare HMO and have a problem with your plan, you should always appeal directly to the plan first. If the plan denies your appeal, the dispute automatically goes to an external reviewer called the Center for Health Dispute Resolution. You will then hear directly from the center.

New Medicare options are now being introduced under the name "Medicare+Choice." Most of these options have no track record, so be wary. If you're happy with the original Medicare, there's no need to change.

People on Medicare should take full advantage of the preventive tests and shots that are given to them free or at low cost. These include:

- Flu vaccine shots
- Pneumococcal vaccine shots
- Screening tests for rectum and colon cancer
- Prostate exams for men (for prostate cancer)
- Mammograms for women (for breast cancer)
- Pap smears for women (for cervical cancer)

Here are good sources of information about Medicare and elder health:

"A SHOPPER'S GUIDE TO LONG-TERM CARE INSURANCE"
NATIONAL ASSOCIATION OF INSURANCE COMMISSIONERS
Publications Department
2301 McGee, Suite 800
Kansas City, MO 64108-2604
(816) 842-3600
www.naic.org
Free guide recommended by Medicare.

AARP
601 E Street, NW
Washington, DC 20049
Member Services: (800) 424-3410
To join: (800) 898-7511
National Headquarters: (202) 434-2277
www.aarp.org
A member services organization for people 50 and over, providing a wide range of programs. Members can purchase hospital indemnity, Medicare supplement, and long-term-care insurance. The insurance plans from AARP are very popular.

ELDERCARE LOCATOR
(800) 677-1116
Call for information on senior services in your community.

HEALTH CARE FINANCING ADMINISTRATION (HCFA)
7500 Security Boulevard
Baltimore, MD 21244
(410) 786-3000
www.hcfa.gov
This is the government agency that oversees Medicare and other government health programs. It has a very good web site.

HENRY J. KAISER FAMILY FOUNDATION
2400 Sand Hill Road
Menlo Park, CA 94025
Publications Line: (800) 656-4533
www.kff.org
Offers a free booklet titled "Talking with Your Parents about Medicare and Health Coverage."

HOSPICE EDUCATION INSTITUTE
190 Westbrook Road
Essex, CT 06426-1510
(800) 331-1620
www.hospiceworld.org
A not-for-profit organization that runs the Hospice Link hotline, which refers callers to local hospice programs and provides information about hospice care.

HOSPICE FOUNDATION OF AMERICA
2001 S Street NW, Suite 300
Washington, DC 20009
(800) 854-3402
www.hospicefoundation.org
A not-for-profit organization that provides free information and education about hospices, grief, and bereavement.

MEDICARE FRAUD HOTLINE
U.S. Department of Health and Human Services
Office of the Inspector General
(800) 447-8477
Medicare fraud costs all of us, from Medicare recipients to taxpayers. If you have evidence of fraud, contact this hotline. You may receive a reward if your tip uncovers fraud.

MEDICARE RIGHTS CENTER
1460 Broadway, 11th floor
New York, NY 10036
(212) 869-3850
www.medicarerights.org
"Established in 1989, Medicare Rights Center is the only national, not-for-profit organization exclusively devoted to ensuring that seniors and people with disabilities on Medicare have access to quality, affordable health care." Services include telephone hotline counseling, seminars and other public education, a Medicare Assistance Plan, publications, and advocacy.

MEDICARE WEB SITE
www.medicare.gov
You can use the Medicare Compare database to find a list of Medicare managed-care plans offered in your area.

MEDIGAP INFORMATION
Check Medigap policies for free, online, at www.quotesmith.com
and other insurance web sites.
Weiss Ratings, (800) 289-9222, will mail you a list of Medigap
policies in your area for $49.

NATIONAL COUNCIL ON THE AGING
409 Third Street SW, Suite 200
Washington, DC 20024
(800) 424-9046
www.ncoa.org
Provides free information, including booklets on different diseases.

NATIONAL HEALTH LAW PROGRAM
2639 S. La Cienega Boulevard
Los Angeles, CA 90034
(310) 204-6010
www.healthlaw.org
Provides advocacy for the elderly, poor, and disabled.

NATIONAL MEDICARE HOTLINE
(800) MEDICARE
Information and assistance for Medicare recipients.

NATIONAL SOCIAL SECURITY HOTLINE
(800) 772-1213

UNITED SENIORS HEALTH COOPERATIVE
409 Third Street SW, Suite 200
Washington, DC 20024-3212
(800) 637-2604
www.ushc-online.org
Provides a book called Long-Term-Care Planning: A Dollars
and Cents Guide *for $18.50.*

Strategies for Saving Money on Health Coverage Used by Individuals and Self-Employed People

One in six Americans have no health insurance coverage whatsoever—and the numbers are growing. A quarter of these people are children. Yet finding affordable individual coverage is very difficult. To help, this section summarizes strategies for individuals who want to get the most reasonable coverage possible.

You can start by contacting the insurance companies and HMOs in your area to inquire about individual health plans. These plans are often available, but quite expensive. Then look into getting a better price by joining a group health plan. Even if you're self-employed, you may be able to find coverage through an association, union, or other group of which you become a member.

Look into government programs. If you have a very low income, or if you have exhausted all of your financial resources because of a health crisis, you're probably eligible for Medicaid. Call your local Medicaid office. As we said earlier, you should not feel ashamed to go on a government-sponsored health program. You have been paying taxes to support these programs for years. If you have children, they are probably eligible for coverage even if you're not—and no child should lack health care.

Internet sites where you can buy health insurance are popping up regularly. The sites claim to make it easy to buy inexpensive health insurance along with other types of insurance coverage. From what we've seen, these services are still spotty and incomplete, offering plans only from a small number of companies in limited geographical areas. The sites may turn into useful resources in the future, but for now investigate their claims thoroughly.

If you're leaving a job where you had health coverage, you are probably entitled to at least 18 additional months of the same coverage under COBRA. Speak to the employee benefits person before you leave the job. As we said earlier, COBRA is usually the best deal you will find.

Alternatively, you could look into setting up a Medical Savings Account (MSA). This is a new approach to paying for health care that allows you to put pretax dollars into an account and use the funds to pay for a wide range of health care expenses, with the balance working as an investment vehicle. MSAs are complicated and controversial, so you should speak with a benefits counselor or investment advisor. Many health care advocates dislike MSAs. Mark Scherzer, a New York health care attorney, says, "MSAs threaten the integrity of the insurance system by removing higher paid and healthier consumers from the premium-paying group."

Finally, a word to those people who choose not to get health coverage because they just don't feel like paying the monthly premiums. We're not going to warn you about getting hit by that bus, because we know that you think you're invulnerable and immortal. We'll just say this: Your parents are worried about your health, and they're also concerned about being forced into bankruptcy by your hospital bills. We know. They call us.

Free Resources on the Internet

There are now more than 20,000 health-related web sites, with new ones launched every day. The Internet has emerged as an excellent resource of information about health care. A majority of Internet users have searched online for health questions.

As much as anything else, the Internet has the power to reshape, and improve, our health care system. The smartest people we know have spoken of their great hopes for the Internet and its ability to deliver health information and human interaction.

According to expert Ellen Severoni, "Improving health

care is not one discussion, it's many discussions that are ongo-
ing over time. I think we're getting there, and the Internet will
help. I'm the least technical person in the world, but I do think
that the Internet is going to level all of the barriers we have,
because it will provide people with so much information."

As with everything else on the Internet, be skeptical about
medical claims and "breakthroughs." It's just as easy for a
quack to set up a web site as it is for a brilliant doctor or cutting-edge medical researcher. Check to see if a site includes a
statement of ownership and funding (with a discussion of
potential conflicts of interest), author biographies, identification of citations, and dates for its postings.

Confidentiality is a serious issue. Be wary about giving
your medical information to anyone online. A survey released
in February 2000 by the California HealthCare Foundation
showed that many health sites fail to protect consumer confidentiality. Even those sites which post strong confidentiality
policies often do not carry through on them. They commonly
"share information" with third parties, including marketing
firms which gather data on huge numbers of individuals and
households.

We encourage you to do research about your conditions on
the Internet. If you see something on the Internet that you
would like to discuss with your doctor, first evaluate its source.
When patients bring in articles from unknown or untrustwor-
thy sources, doctors can become impatient and even defensive.
If you read an article on a reliable news site that tells you about
a study published in a medical journal, go to the site of that
journal and print out the original article to bring to your doctor. The most reliable sources of medical information are the
Journal of the American Medical Association, the *New
England Journal of Medicine, The Lancet,* and the National
Institutes of Health.

Here are some of the better web sites. Additional web sites
are listed under specific subject areas in this book.

For more information about our books and projects, check out our web site at **www.LernerHealth.com.**

AMA HEALTH INSIGHT
www.ama-assn.org/consumer.htm
Information for health consumers prepared by the American Medical Association.

ASK DR. WEIL
www.drweil.com
A site that focuses on alternative and complementary health care.

CANCERNET
cancernet.nci.nih.gov
A site from the National Cancer Institute that has resources for patients, researchers, and health professionals.

CENTER FOR ALTERNATIVE MEDICINE RESEARCH
UNIVERSITY OF TEXAS
www.sph.uth.tmc.edu/utcam/default.htm
A site for an NIH-affiliated center dedicated to "investigating the effectiveness of alternative/complementary therapies used for cancer prevention and control."

CENTERWATCH
www.centerwatch.com
Lists thousands of current clinical trials, along with newly approved drug therapies.

CLINICAL TRIALS
www.clinicaltrials.gov
A site from the National Institutes of Health that lists thousands of clinical trials.

CNN HEALTH NEWS
www.cnn.com/health
Health news stories from the Cable News Network.

CONSUMER REPORTS ONLINE
www.ConsumerReports.org
The online service of the nation's premier consumer magazine. Some parts of the web site are free, but others require a subscription ($24 for a year, $19 for current magazine subscribers, or by a monthly charge).

CONSUMER'S CHECKBOOK
www.checkbook.org
*A not-for-profit organization that provides fee-based
information about top doctors and hospitals.*

DRKOOP.COM
www.drkoop.com
*A source of health information approved by respected
former Surgeon General Dr. C. Everett Koop.*

DRUG INFONET
www.druginfonet.com
*Extensive information, including package inserts, on popular
pharmaceutical drugs, along with contact information
for drug companies.*

GO ASK ALICE
COLUMBIA UNIVERSITY HEALTH SERVICE
www.goaskalice.columbia.edu
*A web site for young women and men about physical and emotional
health.*

HEALTH CARE FINANCING ADMINISTRATION
www.hcfa.gov
*The site of the government agency that administers Medicare,
Medicaid, and Child Health Insurance Programs.*

HEALTH ON THE NET FOUNDATION
www.hon.ch
*A not-for-profit organization based in Geneva, Switzerland that
gives a seal of approval to health web sites meeting its criteria.*

HEALTHFINDER
www.healthfinder.gov
*A government-run site that helps you find useful
health information.*

HEALTHWEB
www.healthweb.org
A good search engine for health information.

HENRY J. KAISER FAMILY FOUNDATION
www.kff.org
*Provides extensive information about health
policy issues.*

INSTITUTE FOR HEALTH CARE RESEARCH AND POLICY
GEORGETOWN UNIVERSITY
www.georgetown.edu/research/ihcrp/hipaa
Explains consumer health care rights in all 50 states.

INSURANCE NEWS NETWORK
www.insure.com
*Lists ratings of the financial strength of insurers and
managed-care companies, and provides other insurance
information.*

INTELIHEALTH
www.intelihealth.com
*An online health publisher in partnership with
Johns Hopkins Medical Center.*

INTERNATIONAL BIBLIOGRAPHIC INFORMATION ON
DIETARY SUPPLEMENTS
www.nal.usda.gov/fnic/IBIDS
*This site from the National Institutes of Health includes
extensive information on supplements and herbal products.*

IVILLAGE
www.ivillage.com
*A leading web site for and about women. It has an
extensive health section.*

JOURNAL OF THE AMERICAN MEDICAL ASSOCIATION
www.amapublications.com
The online version of the prestigious medical journal.

THE LANCET
www.thelancet.com
The web site of the leading British medical journal.

MAYO CLINIC HEALTH OASIS
www.mayohealth.org
*Provides information about a range of illnesses, from
doctors at the famed clinic.*

MEDICINENET
www.medicinenet.com
*Information on medical care prepared by doctors for a
general audience.*

MEDICONSULT
www.mediconsult.com
A site with extensive medical information.

MEDI-NET
www.askmedi.com
A commercial service that will give you extensive information about almost any doctor for $14.75 per report.

MEDSCAPE
www.medscape.com
Search thousands of medical papers and news stories on this site geared to doctors.

NATIONAL CANCER INSTITUTE
www.nci.nih.gov
Information about cancer for patients and researchers.

NATIONAL CENTER FOR COMPLEMENTARY AND
    ALTERNATIVE MEDICINE
nccam.nih.gov
An informative resource on alternative medicine from the National Institutes of Health.

NATIONAL CLEARINGHOUSE FOR ALCOHOL AND
    DRUG INFORMATION
www.health.org/index.htm
Information about drug abuse and prevention.

NATIONAL GUIDELINE CLEARINGHOUSE
www.guideline.org
Gives authoritative treatment guidelines for a range of conditions.

NATIONAL INSTITUTES OF HEALTH
www.nih.gov
Useful information, including lists of government-funded studies of many diseases.

NATIONAL ORGANIZATION FOR RARE DISORDERS
www.rarediseases.org
Information and support for people with little-known diseases.

NEW ENGLAND JOURNAL OF MEDICINE
www.nejm.org
Provides information from the medical journal.

ONCOLINK
www.oncolink.upenn.edu
A cancer site for patients and doctors from the University of Pennsylvania.

ONHEALTH
www.OnHealth.com
A commercial web site with health information for women.

PUBMED
www.ncbi.nlm.nih.gov/PubMed
Provides abstracts (summaries of articles) from thousands of medical journals in the National Library of Medicine, along with helpful consumer information.

QUACKWATCH
www.quackwatch.com
A useful and often funny site that exposes fraudulent and deceptive health care practices.

RAND
www.rand.org
You can obtain many reports and studies on health care issues for little or no cost from the web site of this well-known think tank.

REUTERS HEALTH INFORMATION
www.reutershealth.com
A health information service of the international news operation.

ROBERT WOOD JOHNSON FAMILY FOUNDATION
www.rwjf.org
Provides information about health policy issues.

SENIORNET
www.seniornet.com
A not-for-profit web site for and about seniors.

SUPPLEMENT TESTING INSTITUTE
www.supplementtesting.org
An independent organization that approves dietary supplements that have passed quality and potency tests.

THE BODY: AN AIDS AND HIV INFORMATION RESOURCE
www.thebody.com
A site with extensive information for people affected by HIV and AIDS.

USDA
www.usda.gov
*Information on food and diet from the U.S. Department
of Agriculture.*

WebMD
www.webmd.com
A large and popular commercial health site.

Wellness Web
www.wellweb.com
*Extensive information on alternative health, including herbs,
supplements, and nutrition, as well as conventional medicine.*

7.

Preventing Health Problems

"He who has health has hope, and he who has hope has everything."

— ARAB PROVERB

Prevention Works

THERE IS NOW A GREATER APPRECIATION THAN EVER THAT health prevention works. By exercising regularly, not smoking, eating nutritiously, and taking good care of yourself, you will likely live a longer and healthier life. By taking advantage of free physical exams and health programs, you will get a big boost toward living that healthy lifestyle.

Managed care has its drawbacks, but one of its best features is an emphasis on prevention. Take advantage of every free and low-cost program and screening offered by your health plan. Common tests include mammography (to check for breast cancer), pap smears (for cervical cancer), prostate tests (for prostate cancer), x-rays, and blood tests. Popular programs include smoking cessation, weight loss, fitness and diet workshops, managing your blood pressure, well child care, stress prevention, and health education seminars.

Regular physicals present an excellent opportunity not

only to get a checkup, but also to set goals for exercise and diet, develop a stronger relationship with your doctor, and learn more about the services you're entitled to receive under your health plan. Every time you add to your knowledge of medicine in general and your own body in particular, you make a positive step towards living a long and healthy life.

Doctors recognize the importance of lifestyle issues, but sometimes feel too rushed to discuss them during appointments. Tell your doctor you want to discuss these issues. People would rather get advice on health risk behaviors from their doctor than from anyone else, according to a recent survey.

Don't let denial stop you from taking advantage of prevention programs. Recently we gave a talk where one audience member discussed his health situation. He was looking to join a health plan because for the last 25 years he had carried only a hospitalization plan. He had not been hospitalized in that entire time. When we congratulated him on his good health, he responded, "But I've never had a physical exam in all those years. I'm scared of what they will find when I do finally go to a doctor."

Don't scare yourself to death. Take positive steps for health now.

Our Patient's Bill of Responsibilities

Throughout this book, we have recommended that you be an informed and assertive consumer of health care, and that you be ready to speak up for your rights.

We believe that patients have responsibilities, too.

1. Treat doctors, nurses, hospital staff, health plan employees, and other medical personnel with respect. Being assertive (and sometimes even "difficult") doesn't mean being rude and obnoxious. Some medical personnel are unpleasant and lacking in bedside manner. Then again,

they have to deal with some patients who are hostile because illness has made them angry, depressed, or disoriented.

2. Take your medications and follow your treatment regimens. Treatment decisions can be made jointly, by you and your doctor. Once these decisions are made, you have a responsibility to follow them. Some patients refuse to take their medications or follow treatment regimens, and wind up with worse health problems needing greater medical attention. If you start a treatment but feel it's not working, don't just stop. Contact your doctor to discuss alternatives.

3. Educate yourself. Learn everything that you can about the condition or illness confronting you or a loved one.

4. Take control of your own care. Tell your doctors and other health care professionals that you want to be an active partner in your treatment, and follow through.

5. Talk to your loved ones and make your wishes known. In addition to a will, write up a health care proxy and a living will. These documents will help you get what you need when you are incapacitated and unable to express your wishes. If you have already completed these documents, make certain to update them as your needs change. Keep all the documents in one easy-to-find place.

Good Living, Good Health

We have written about the responsibilities of health plans, doctors, hospitals, and the health care system, and have provided you with information and strategies so that you can get the best health care for yourself and your loved ones.

One fact remains: The person most responsible for your

health is *you*. Yes, Julie's getting cancer at the age of 26 was a shocking development that none of us could have predicted. And yes, any one of us could get hit by that proverbial bus.

Still, we are fortunate to live in a time of medical progress and scientific breakthroughs. A child born in the United States today will live, on average, to be nearly 77. The fastest-growing part of our society is the elderly—many of whom are leading very active lives. Our grandmother, Rose Lerner, to whom this book is dedicated, recently celebrated her 96th birthday.

Many people die of preventable illnesses brought on by decades of unwise lifestyle choices. Each year, unhealthy lifestyle behaviors cost our country $200 billion in health expenditures. More than 40% of deaths are related to unhealthy behaviors.

We encourage you to live the longest and healthiest life possible, with the fewest visits to doctors and hospitals, by making wise choices. Here's our Top 10 list for staying healthy and living a long and good life:

1. Exercise regularly;
2. Don't smoke or chew tobacco;
3. Eat healthfully, with lots of fruits, vegetables, and whole grains every day;
4. Drink alcohol only in moderation;
5. Learn about safer sex;
6. Get enough sleep;
7. Reduce stress;
8. Drink plenty of water;
9. Drive safely and wear seatbelts;
10. Stay active and involved.

These proven health habits will help you to live longer and save money. Dr. Bob Arnot of NBC News estimates that by taking good care of your own health, you can cut yearly health care costs by as much as a third. Be suspicious of anyone who tells you that you will become "miraculously" healthy just by taking a pill, buying a supplement, or purchasing a fad health book. Bacon will not make you thin—really!

We're not going to go into greater detail about healthy behaviors for one simple reason: you already know what we would say. When we discuss healthy lifestyles with people, we rarely hear ignorance—but we often hear denial.

Why do so many people go on high-fat/high-protein diets to lose weight? Why do some people continue smoking and refuse to exercise, but still claim they're in great shape because they take a lot of vitamins? Why would individuals jump from diet to diet, and supplement to supplement, rather than eating balanced and nutritious meals? They know better—but they're vainly searching for an easy way out.

We understand that it can be hard to eat right and exercise regularly. Still, we've seen many people who have courageously fought life-threatening illnesses and chronic conditions. So we have little patience for those who embrace fads and gimmicks.

If you have questions about diet, exercise, or healthy living, we strongly encourage you to speak with your doctor. There are also many excellent books, magazines, and web sites that can provide you with answers and ideas. But mostly we say: Get over your denial. If you want to live a healthy life, then take the steps that have been proven to result in greater health, fitness, and longevity.

Did you know that volunteering, helping others, and maintaining strong social connections have been shown to improve your health? Many people have learned that when you give to others, you get much more back in return. The not-for-profit service organizations in your community could benefit from your time. By volunteering at a health organization, you will not only feel good, you may also learn about new medical developments which will benefit you and your family.

We'll add another tip. This is something that both of us

have found invaluable. Keep your sense of humor. Through cancer, AIDS, and issues of all kinds, we've seen that being able to laugh at ourselves (and sometimes others) is one of the best things you can do for your health. Keep finding the humor in life and telling jokes. Laughter is not trivial. On the contrary, quite often there is nothing more profound than laughter.

From our family to yours, we wish you and your loved ones the very best of health.

Bonus List: Top 15 Tips for Getting the Best Health Care

1. Recognize that health care is a business and you're a consumer—so be an informed and assertive consumer!

2. If you have a problem with your health plan, first complain directly to the plan. Every health plan has a complaint procedure in place.

3. Whenever you have a problem with a health care company or organization, make your complaint in writing. Send the letter by certified mail with a return receipt requested so that you have a record. Document all phone calls you make (date, time, who you spoke to, what they said). Keep all of your paperwork in one easily accessible place.

4. If your complaint is denied, you can appeal—and you should appeal immediately. Often a company will give in when it recognizes that you're willing to press the matter. Don't be passive.

5. If you receive health coverage through work, get your company's employee benefits people on your side. The company spends far more money buying coverage than you do—and health care administrators will listen carefully to what it says.

6. If you are not happy with the way you are being treated, contact the state health department, insurance department, or Attorney General's office. You can contact state agencies at any time, even just to ask for information.

7. In the hospital, if you or a loved one are having problems, contact the hospital's patient representatives. They will

lobby for you. If you continue to have problems, call the hospital's CEO and demand better treatment.

8. Know your legal rights to health care and demand to get what you deserve.

9. Don't let insurance bureaucrats and health care workers confuse you with insurance lingo or medical jargon. You are the customer—and they should speak in your language.

10. If you have problems, document, complain, and appeal! Demand excellent care, and you're much more likely to get it.

11. If problems continue, call your elected officials and ask them to intercede on your behalf. You can also call the media if you're willing to have your health condition discussed in public. Health care companies are very concerned about political pressure and bad publicity.

12. Find allies in the health system. If your doctor has been supportive, ask her to help you in any conflicts with your health plan or hospital. Get other advocates on your side.

13. Read your health plan's member handbook. We know, we know, it's really boring—but you need to understand what's covered and what's not.

14. Don't be intimidated. The health care industry is set up to make patients feel powerless. Why else would we need to wait in a cold examining room wearing nothing but a paper gown? Be assertive, and don't let anyone intimidate you.

15. Recognize that health care is one of your largest expenses when you include plan premiums, co-payments, deductibles, drugs, medical equipment, and the large portion of your taxes that subsidizes our health system. When you need health care, demand the best—because you have paid for it!

Appendix A:
Health Organizations
That Can Help You

AGENCY FOR HEALTHCARE RESEARCH AND
    QUALITY (AHRQ)
DEPARTMENT OF HEALTH AND HUMAN SERVICES
2101 East Jefferson Street, Suite 600
Rockville, MD 20852
(301) 594-6662
Publications Clearinghouse: (800) 358-9295
www.ahrq.gov
The federal government's think tank on health care issues.

AIDS ACTION COUNCIL
1906 Sunderland Place NW
Washington, DC 20036
(202) 530-8030
www.aidsaction.org
*This council represents more than 3,000 AIDS organizations
from around the nation.*

ALCOHOLICS ANONYMOUS (AA)
Grand Central Station
PO Box 459
New York, NY 10163
(212) 870-3400
www.aa.org
*"A worldwide fellowship of sober alcoholics, whose recovery is
based on Twelve Steps; no dues or fees, self-supporting through
voluntary, small contributions of members, accepts no outside funds;
not affiliated with any other organization; our primary purpose: to
carry the AA message to the alcoholic who still suffers."*

Alliance for Health Reform
1900 L Street NW, Suite 512
Washington, DC 20036
(202) 466-5626
www.allhealth.org
An organization that distributes position papers and provides objective information to decision-makers about the U.S. health care system.

Alliance of Claims Assistance
    Professionals (ACAP)
731 Naperville Road
Wheaton, IL 60187-6407
(630) 588-1260
(877) 275-8765
www.claims.org
An association that helps people find fee-based medical-claims-assistance professionals who can handle health care bills and paperwork.

American Accreditation HealthCare
    Commission/URAC
1275 K Street NW, Suite 1100
Washington, DC 20005
(202) 216-9010
www.urac.org
"A not-for-profit entity founded in 1990 to establish accreditation standards for managed health care organizations."

American Anorexia Bulimia
    Association, Inc.
165 West 46th Street, Suite 1108
New York, NY 10036
(212) 575-6200
www.aabainc.org
A group that provides information, referrals, and educational research on anorexia, bulimia, and other eating disorders.

American Association of Health Plans (AAHP)
1129 20th Street NW, Suite 600
Washington, DC 20036-3421
(202) 778-3200
www.aahp.org
An association that represents more than 1,000 HMOs, PPOs, and other network-based plans with close to 140 million members.

AMERICAN CANCER SOCIETY (ACS)
1599 Clifton Road NE
Atlanta, GA 30329
(800) ACS-2345
www.cancer.org
A leading nationwide organization focused on cancer-related issues.

AMERICAN DIABETES ASSOCIATION
1701 North Beauregard Street
Alexandria, VA 22311
(800) DIABETES
www.diabetes.org
A leading nationwide organization that provides information and services for people with diabetes.

AMERICAN DIETETIC ASSOCIATION
216 West Jackson, Suite 800
Chicago, IL 60606
(312) 899-0040
www.eatright.org
A professional association of dieticians. It provides nutritional information and referrals to its members.

AMERICAN FOUNDATION FOR AIDS RESEARCH
   (AMFAR)
120 Wall Street, 13th floor
New York, NY 10005
(212) 806-1600
www.amfar.org
A national organization that promotes and funds AIDS research.

AMERICAN FOUNDATION FOR SUICIDE PREVENTION
   (AFSP)
120 Wall Street, 22nd floor
New York, NY 10005
(888) 333-2377
www.afsp.org
A foundation that sponsors educational programs and research on suicide.

American Health Information Management
   Association
919 Michigan Avenue
Chicago, IL 60611
(312) 233-1100
www.ahima.org
*A trade association for claims processors. To find someone who can
help you with insurance claims in your city, call and ask for the
Professional Practice Area. Its web site has good information on
keeping your health records.*

American Heart Association (AHA)
7272 Greenville Avenue
Dallas, TX 75231
National Hotline: (800) AHA-USA1
www.americanheart.org
*A leading nationwide organization that works to prevent heart
disease and stroke.*

American Holistic Medical Association (AHMA)
6728 Old McLean Village Drive
McLean, VA 22101
(703) 556-9728
www.holisticmedicine.org
*An association for doctors interested in holistic medicine that provides
information and a "holistic doctor finder."*

American Hospital Association (AHA)
1 North Franklin
Chicago, IL 60606
(312) 422-3000
www.aha.org
An association representing nearly 5,000 hospitals around the nation.

American Lyme Disease Foundation, Inc. (ALDF)
293 Route 100
Somers, NY 10589
(800) 876-5963
www.aldf.com
*A national not-for-profit organization that provides information
and supports research on Lyme disease and other
tick-borne infections.*

AMERICAN MEDICAL ASSOCIATION (AMA)
515 North State Street
Chicago, IL 60610
(312) 464-5000
www.ama-assn.org
The leading trade association representing doctors.

AMERICAN PSYCHIATRIC ASSOCIATION
1400 K Street NW
Washington, DC 20005
(202) 682-6000
www.psych.org
The major association of psychiatrists.

AMERICAN PSYCHOLOGICAL ASSOCIATION
750 First Street NE
Washington, DC 20002-4242
(202) 336-5500
www.apa.org
The major association of psychologists.

ARTHRITIS FOUNDATION
1330 West Peachtree Street
Atlanta, GA 30309
(404) 872-7100
Arthritis Answers: (800) 283-7800
www.arthritis.org
A leading nationwide organization that provides information about arthritis and referrals to local resources.

ARTISTS' HEALTH INSURANCE RESOURCE CENTER
(AHIRC)
Actor's Fund of America
729 Seventh Avenue, 10th floor
New York, NY 10019
(800) 798-8447
www.actorsfund.org/ahirc
A center that offers free resources to help people in the arts community obtain low-cost health insurance.

Business Roundtable (BRT)
1615 L Street NW
Washington, DC 20036
(202) 872-1260
www.brt.org
An organization representing large corporations which also coordinates the Leapfrog Group, an effort to improve health care and reduce medical mistakes.

California Health Decisions
    (CHD)
505 South Main Street, Suite 400
Orange, CA 92868
(714) 647-4922
www.cahd.org
"Founded in 1985, CHD is an independent, nonprofit organization that identifies and communicates public values on issues related to healthcare."

Cancer Care
275 Seventh Avenue, 22nd floor
New York, NY 10001
National Counseling Line: (800) 813-HOPE
www.cancercare.org
A national not-for-profit organization that helps people with cancer, their families and professional caregivers through one-to-one counseling, educational programs, and telephone contact. Also publishes a useful resource guide.

CareCheck.com
2448 East 81st Street, Suite 4040
Tulsa, OK 74137
(877) 642-2100
www.CareCheck.com
A fee-based commercial service which helps people find nursing homes, assisted living facilities, and retirement communities for aging relatives.

Center for Health Care Rights
520 S. Lafayette Park Place, Suite 214
Los Angeles, CA 90057
(213) 383-4519
www.healthcarerights.org
"The Center for Health Care Rights is a non-profit health

care consumer advocacy organization serving consumers through a combination of direct service programs and policy level advocacy. The Center seeks to educate health care consumers on how to advocate for themselves, and seeks to improve the delivery of quality health care through an array of research programs and policy level advocacy." The Center's excellent web site features numerous sample letters and other useful material.

CENTER FOR PATIENT ADVOCACY
1350 Beverly Road, Suite 108
McLean, VA 22101
(703) 748-0400
Free patient hotline: (800) 846-7444
www.patientadvocacy.org
"At the forefront of the battle to ensure that patients have timely access to the highest quality health care in the world."

CENTERS FOR DISEASE CONTROL AND PREVENTION (CDCP)
1600 Clifton Road NE
Atlanta, GA 30333
(404) 639-3311
(800) 311-3435
www.cdc.gov
An agency of the federal government; its mission is "to promote health and quality of life by preventing and controlling disease, injury, and disability."

CHILDREN'S DEFENSE FUND
25 E Street NW
Washington, DC 20001
(202) 628-8787
www.childrensdefense.org
Advocates for health insurance for all children, among other issues.

CHOICE IN DYING
1035 30th Street NW
Washington, DC 20007
(202) 338-9790
Counseling Hotline: (800) 989-9455
www.choices.org
An advocacy group for the right to die. Provides forms for living wills and health care proxies.

Consumer Coalition for Quality
    Health Care
1275 K Street NW, Suite 602
Washington, DC 20005
(202) 789-3606
Quality Watchline: (800) 720-8090
www.consumers.org
*A not-for-profit consortium of organizations which advocates for
health care access.*

Consumers for Quality Care
1750 Ocean Park Boulevard, Suite 200
Santa Monica, CA 90405
(310) 392-0522
www.consumerwatchdog.org
*"A project of the Foundation for Taxpayer and Consumer Rights estab-
lished in 1994 to investigate and report publicly on the epidemic of
medical malpractice and reckless corporate care-cutting by HMOs."*

Consumers Union (CU)
101 Truman Avenue
Yonkers, NY 10703
(914) 378-2000
www.ConsumersUnion.org
www.ConsumerReports.org
*"Consumers Union is a nonprofit membership organization
chartered in 1936 under the laws of the State of New York to
provide consumers with information, education, and counsel about
goods, services, health, and personal finance; and to initiate and
cooperate with individual and group efforts to maintain and
enhance the quality of life for consumers. Consumers Union's
income is solely derived from the sale of* Consumer Reports, *its
other publications and services, and from noncommercial
contributions, grants, and fees. In addition to reports on Consumers
Union's own product testing,* Consumer Reports *with approximately
5 million paid circulation, regularly carries articles on health,
product safety, marketplace economics, and legislative, judicial,
and regulatory actions which affect consumer welfare. Consumers
Union's publications and services carry no outside advertising and
receive no commercial support. Consumers Union has long
advocated on behalf of the interests of consumers in the delivery
of health care, including advocacy on the issues of delivery
of health care services through managed care."*

COUNCIL ON FAMILY HEALTH (CFH)
1155 Connecticut Avenue NW, Suite 400
Washington, DC 20036
(202) 429-6600
www.cfhinfo.org
*The Council educates consumers about health and safety issues, includ-
ing the proper use of prescription and nonprescription medicines.*

CURE FOR LYMPHOMA FOUNDATION (CFL)
215 Lexington Avenue
New York, NY 10016
(212) 213-9595
(800) CFL-6848
www.cfl.org
*"A nationwide not-for-profit foundation dedicated to funding research,
providing information, and supporting those whose lives have been
touched by Hodgkin's disease and non-Hodgkin's lymphoma."*

ECRI
5200 Butler Pike
Plymouth Meeting, PA 19462-1298
(610) 825-6000
www.ecri.org
*A not-for-profit health services research agency that works with
the World Health Organization and the Agency for Healthcare
Research and Quality. Among its many activities, ECRI provides
studies on medical devices, drugs, and surgical procedures.*

EMPLOYEE BENEFIT RESEARCH INSTITUTE (EBRI)
2121 K Street NW, Suite 600
Washington, DC 20037-1896
(202) 659-0670
www.ebri.org
*EBRI is a leading think tank on employee benefits issues that
functions "strictly in an objective and unbiased manner and
not as an advocate or opponent of any position."*

FAMILIES USA
1334 G Street NW
Washington, DC 20005
(202) 628-3030
www.familiesusa.org
*"Families USA is a national non-profit, non-partisan organization
dedicated to the achievement of high-quality affordable health and
long-term care for all Americans."*

Federal Consumer Information Center (FCIC)
PO Box 100
Pueblo, CO 81009
(888) 8-PUEBLO
www.pueblo.gsa.gov
*This center offers free and low-cost booklets from federal
agencies on health, children, food, government programs,
and other topics.*

Foundation for Accountability (FACCT)
520 SW Sixth Avenue, Suite 700
Portland, OR 97204
(503) 223-2228
www.facct.org
*"A not-for-profit organization dedicated to helping Americans make
better health care decisions," with a focus on defining health care quality.*

Foundation for the Advancement of
    Innovative Medicine (FAIM)
485 Kinderkamack Road, 2nd floor
Oradell, NJ 07649
(877) 634-3246
www.faim.org
*The Foundation "provides awareness, education, and activism
in the area of complementary medicine."*

Health Care Financing Administration (HCFA)
7500 Security Boulevard
Baltimore, MD 21244
(410) 786-3000
www.hcfa.gov
*HCFA administers the Medicare, Medicaid, and Child Health
Insurance Programs, paying the medical bills for more than
75 million beneficiaries.*

Health Insurance Association of America (HIAA)
555 13th Street NW, Suite 600 East
Washington, DC 20004
(202) 824-1600
www.hiaa.org
*"The nation's leading trade association for the private, for-profit
health insurance industry." Its 290 members provide health,
long-term care, dental, disability, and supplemental coverage to
more than 123 million Americans.*

HENRY J. KAISER FAMILY FOUNDATION (KFF)
2400 Sand Hill Road
Menlo Park, CA 94025
(650) 854-9400
www.kff.org
"An independent health care philanthropy focusing on major health care issues facing the nation."

HUNTINGTON'S DISEASE SOCIETY OF AMERICA (HDSA)
158 West 29th Street, 7th floor
New York, NY 10001-5300
(212) 242-1968
(800) 345-HDSA
www.hdsa.org
A national organization devoted to the care and cure of Huntington's disease.

HYSTERECTOMY EDUCATIONAL RESOURCES AND
    SERVICES FOUNDATION (HERS)
422 Bryn Mawr Avenue
Bala Cynwyd, PA 19004
(610) 667-7757
www.ccon.com/hers
"The HERS Foundation is an independent non-profit national and international women's health education organization. It provides full, accurate information about hysterectomy, its adverse effects and alternative treatments."

INDEPENDENT INSURANCE AGENTS OF AMERICA
    (IIAA)
127 South Peyton Street
Alexandria, VA 22314
(800) 221-7917
www.independentagent.com
An association representing independent insurance agents. Its web site provides information on finding an independent agent.

INTERNATIONAL CHIROPRACTORS ASSOCIATION
1110 N. Glebe Road, Suite 1000
Arlington, VA 22201
(800) 423-4690
www.chiropractic.org
An association that provides information and referrals to chiropractors.

Joint Commission on Accreditation of
   Healthcare Organizations (JCAHO)
1 Renaissance Boulevard
Oakbrook Terrace, IL 60181
(630) 792-5000
www.jcaho.org
JCAHO accredits more than 18,000 hospitals and health care
organizations and programs in the United States.

Juvenile Diabetes Foundation (JDF)
120 Wall Street, 19th floor
New York, NY 10005
(800) JDF-CURE
www.jdf.org
"JDF is the world's leading nonprofit, nongovernmental funder of
diabetes research. Founded in 1970 by parents of children
with diabetes, JDF's mission is to find a cure for diabetes and
its complications through the support of research."

Kushi Institute
PO Box 7
Becket, MA 01223
(413) 623-5741
(800) 975-8744
www.kushiinstitute.org
A leading macrobiotic educational center founded in 1978.

La Leche League International
1400 N. Meacham Road
Schaumburg, IL 60173-4048
(847) 519-7730
(800) 525-3243
www.lalecheleague.org
An international not-for-profit organization that provides information
and support on breastfeeding and the mothering experience.

Lamaze International
1200 19th Street NW, Suite 300
Washington, DC 20036-2422
(202) 857-1128
(800) 368-4404
www.lamaze-childbirth.com
"The Lamaze mission is to promote normal, natural, healthy, and
fulfilling childbearing experiences for women and their families
through education, advocacy, and reform."

LEUKEMIA & LYMPHOMA SOCIETY
600 Third Avenue, 4th floor
New York, NY 10016
(212) 450-8888
Information Resource Center: (800) 955-4572
www.leukemia.org
Formerly the Leukemia Society of America, this not-for-profit
organization provides free services to people affected by leukemia
and lymphoma.

MARCH OF DIMES BIRTH DEFECTS FOUNDATION
1275 Mamaroneck Avenue
White Plains, NY 10605
(914) 428-7100
Resource Center: (888) 663-4637
www.modimes.org
President Franklin D. Roosevelt started the organization to fight polio;
now its mission is "to improve the health of babies by preventing birth
defects and infant mortality."

MUSCULAR DYSTROPHY ASSOCIATION (MDA)
3300 E. Sunrise Drive
Tucson, AZ 85718
(520) 529-2000
www.mdausa.org
A voluntary organization that provides free services for people
with muscular dystrophy.

NATIONAL ACADEMY OF ELDER LAW ATTORNEYS (NAELA)
1604 North Country Club Road
Tucson, AZ 85716
(520) 881-4005
www.naela.org
A not-for-profit association assisting lawyers and others who
work with older clients and their families.

NATIONAL ALLIANCE FOR THE MENTALLY ILL (NAMI)
Colonial Place Three
2107 Wilson Boulevard, Suite 300
Arlington, VA 22201-3042
(703) 524-7600
Helpline: (800) 950-6264
www.nami.org
"With more than 210,000 members, NAMI is the nation's leading
grassroots advocacy organization solely dedicated to improving the
lives of persons with severe mental illnesses."

NATIONAL ALLIANCE OF BREAST CANCER ORGANIZATIONS
(NABCO)
9 East 37th Street, 10th floor
New York, NY 10016
(212) 889-0606
(888) 806-2226
www.nabco.org
A resource that provides information, assistance, and publications on breast cancer.

NATIONAL ASSOCIATION FOR HOME CARE (NAHC)
228 Seventh Street SE
Washington, DC 20003
(202) 547-7424
www.nahc.org
"NAHC is the nation's largest trade association that represents the interests of home care agencies, hospices, and home care aid organizations."

NATIONAL ASSOCIATION OF INSURANCE
COMMISSIONERS (NAIC)
2301 McGee, Suite 800
Kansas City, MO 64108-2604
(816) 842-3600
www.naic.org
The association of state insurance regulators.

NATIONAL CANCER INSTITUTE (NCI)
Building 31, Room 10A24
9000 Rockville Place
Bethesda, MD 20892
(800) 4-CANCER
www.nci.nih.gov
A government institute that researches cancer and funds other cancer efforts.

NATIONAL CENTER FOR COMPLEMENTARY AND
ALTERNATIVE MEDICINE (NCCAM)
National Institutes of Health
PO Box 8218
Silver Spring, MD 20907-8218
(888) 644-6226
nccam.nih.gov
A center providing information on studies in complementary and alternative medicine, and referrals to other sources of information. (Does not answer medical questions or provide referrals to practitioners.)

THE NATIONAL CENTER ON ADDICTION AND
    SUBSTANCE ABUSE (CASA)
Columbia University Health Sciences Division
152 West 57th Street, 12th floor
New York, NY 10019-3310
(212) 841-5200
www.casacolumbia.org
A leading think tank on issues relating to substance abuse.

NATIONAL CLEARINGHOUSE FOR ALCOHOL AND
    DRUG INFORMATION (NCADI)
PO Box 2345
Rockville, MD 20847
(800) 729-6686
www.health.org
One of the world's largest resources for information and materials
concerning substance abuse, NCADI distributes publications and
provides treatment referrals to community organizations.

NATIONAL COALITION OF MENTAL HEALTH
    PROFESSIONALS & CONSUMERS, INC.
PO Box 438
Commack, NY 11725
(516) 424-5232
(888) SAY-NO-MC
www.nomanagedcare.org
An organization of mental health activists opposed to
managed care.

NATIONAL COMMITTEE FOR QUALITY ASSURANCE
    (NCQA)
2000 L Street NW, Suite 500
Washington, DC 20036
(202) 955-3500
Publications: (800) 839-6487
Customer Support Line: (888) 275-7585
www.ncqa.org
Accredits HMOs and other managed-care organizations. The
accreditation has been somewhat limited in scope, but is steadily
expanding. HMOs are not required to obtain NCQA accreditation,
and only about half go through the process. The NCQA has
limited information on its web site. Additional data is available
for purchase, but the most useful information, called HEDIS,
is very expensive.

NATIONAL DOWN SYNDROME SOCIETY (NDSS)
666 Broadway, Suite 810
New York, NY 10012
(212) 460-9330
(800) 221-4602
www.ndss.org
A national organization that provides services to people with Down syndrome and to their families.

NATIONAL INFORMATION CENTER FOR CHILDREN
    AND YOUTH WITH DISABILITIES (NICHCY)
PO Box 1492
Washington, DC 20013
(800) 695-0285
www.nichcy.org
A government-funded center that provides referrals and free or low-cost publications about children and youth with disabilities.

NATIONAL INSTITUTE OF MENTAL HEALTH (NIMH)
6001 Executive Boulevard, Room 8184, MSC 9663
Bethesda, MD 20892-9663
(301) 443-4513
www.nimh.nih.gov
The mission of NIMH is "to diminish the burden of mental illness through research." Its web site has information on mental-health related events, literature, and clinical trials.

NATIONAL INSTITUTE OF NEUROLOGICAL
    DISORDERS AND STROKE (NINDS)
National Institutes of Health
PO Box 5801
Bethesda, MD 20892
(800) 352-9424
www.ninds.nih.gov
The institute provides information on stroke, Parkinson's disease, epilepsy, migraines, muscular dystrophy, multiple sclerosis, and other disorders.

NATIONAL INSTITUTE ON AGING (NIA)
INFORMATION CENTER
PO Box 8057
Gaithersburg, MD 20898
(800) 222-2225
www.nih.gov/nia
The institute provides information on nursing homes, long-term care, and other aging issues.

NATIONAL MARFAN FOUNDATION
382 Main Street
Port Washington, NY 11050
(800) 8-MARFAN
www.marfan.org
"Serving the needs of people with the Marfan syndrome and related connective tissue disorders."

NATIONAL MATERNAL AND CHILD HEALTH
    CLEARINGHOUSE (NMCHC)
2070 Chain Bridge Road, Suite 450
Vienna, VA 22182
(888) 434-4624
www.nmchc.org
The Clearinghouse provides free materials and referrals about maternal and child health and SIDS.

NATIONAL MENTAL HEALTH ASSOCIATION
    (NMHA)
1021 Prince Street
Alexandria, VA 22314-2971
(800) 969-NMHA
www.nmha.org
A mental health advocacy organization that provides free information and referrals for mental health issues.

NATIONAL MULTIPLE SCLEROSIS SOCIETY (NMSS)
733 Third Avenue
New York, NY 10017
(800) 344-4867
www.nmss.org
NMSS provides free comprehensive support services to help people with MS and their families.

NATIONAL ORGANIZATION FOR RARE DISORDERS
    (NORD)
PO Box 8923
New Fairfield, CT 06812-8923
(203) 746-6518
(800) 999-NORD
www.rarediseases.org
NORD provides patient services, information, education, and advocacy for people affected by rare disorders.

NATIONAL OSTEOPOROSIS FOUNDATION
   (NOF)
1232 22nd Street NW
Washington, DC 20037-1292
(202) 223-2226
www.nof.org
This foundation provides information and education about osteoporosis. It also promotes research on osteoporosis and related bone diseases.

NATIONAL STROKE ASSOCIATION
9707 E. Easter Lane
Englewood, CO 80112-3747
(800) STROKES
www.stroke.org
An association that provides information and referrals for people affected by stroke.

NATIONAL WOMEN'S HEALTH INFORMATION CENTER
U.S. Department of Health and Human Services
8550 Arlington Boulevard, Suite 300
Fairfax, VA 22031
(800) 994-WOMAN
www.4woman.gov
"A one-stop gateway for women seeking health information," the Center provides material and referrals on hundreds of topics in women's health.

NATIONAL WOMEN'S HEALTH NETWORK
514 10th Street NW, Suite 400
Washington, DC 20004
(202) 628-7814
www.womenshealthnetwork.org
"The only national public interest membership-based organization advocating for the health of all U.S. women for nearly twenty-five years."

PARKINSON'S DISEASE FOUNDATION (PDF)
710 West 168th Street
New York, NY 10032-9982
(800) 457-6676
www.pdf.org
This foundation provides information about Parkinson's disease and promotes research into the cause and cure of the illness.

People's Medical Society
462 Walnut Street
Allentown, PA 18102
(800) 624-8773
www.peoplesmed.org
"The largest medical consumer advocacy organization in the United States," this not-for-profit organization publishes consumer-oriented books and other materials about health care.

Planned Parenthood Federation of America, Inc.
810 Seventh Avenue
New York, NY 10019
(212) 541-7800
www.plannedparenthood.org
Teen web site: www.teenwire.com
Planned Parenthood is a nationwide not-for-profit organization focusing on contraceptive and reproductive health, including birth control, family planning, education, HIV testing, sexually transmitted diseases, and counseling.

Project Inform
205 13th Street, Suite 2001
San Francisco, CA 94103
(415) 558-8669
Treatment Options Hotline: (800) 822-7422
www.projectinform.org
An information clearinghouse for HIV information and AIDS treatment options.

Public Citizen
1600 20th Street NW
Washington, DC 20009
(202) 588-1000
www.citizen.org
A not-for-profit citizen's organization which has a well-regarded Health Research Group. It publishes a large book called 16,638 Questionable Doctors. You can order a report on questionable doctors in your state for $23.50. Public Citizen was founded by Ralph Nader in 1971.

RAND
PO Box 2138
Santa Monica, CA 90407
(310) 393-0411
Publications: (310) 451-7002
www.rand.org
A leading think tank on issues including health care. It has numerous reports and studies on health care available for little or no cost.

RESOLVE
1310 Broadway
Somerville, MA 02144
Helpline: (617) 623-0744
www.resolve.org
A not-for-profit organization providing information and support to infertile couples and individuals.

ROBERT WOOD JOHNSON FAMILY FOUNDATION
Route 1 and College Road East
PO Box 2316
Princeton, NJ 08543-2316
(609) 452-8701
www.rwjf.org
This foundation gives grants to organizations in fulfillment of its mission "to improve the health and health care of all Americans."

ROSENTHAL CENTER FOR COMPLEMENTARY AND
ALTERNATIVE MEDICINE
Columbia University
College of Physicians & Surgeons
630 West 168th Street, Box 75
New York, NY 10032
(212) 543-9550
cpmcnet.columbia.edu/dept/rosenthal
The Center's web site has useful fact sheets about alternative medicine, homeopathy, acupuncture, herbal medicine, and other topics.

UNITED WAY OF AMERICA
701 N. Fairfax Street
Alexandria, VA 22314-2045
(703) 836-7100
To find your local chapter: (800) 411-UWAY
www.unitedway.org
United Way chapters are major supporters of local not-for-profit organizations.

Appendix B:

Hotlines and Helplines

Alzheimer's National Association Hotline: (800) 272-3900
American Cancer Society Response Line: (800) ACS-2345
American Council on Alcoholism: (800) 527-5344
American Diabetes Association: (800) DIABETES
American Heart Association: (800) AHA-USA1
Arthritis Answers: (800) 283-7800
Bone Marrow Hotline: (800) LINK-BMT
Cancer Care National Counseling Line: (800) 813-HOPE
CDC Immunization Hotline: (800) 232-7468
CDC Sexually Transmitted Disease Hotline:
     (800) 227-8922
Center for Patient Advocacy Hotline: (800) 846-7444
Child Health Insurance Program (CHIP) Hotline:
     (877) KIDS-NOW
Choice in Dying Counseling Hotline: (800) 989-9455
Cocaine Anonymous Helpline: (212) 262-2463
FDA Consumer Hotline: (888) INFO-FDA
Hospice Link: (800) 331-1620
La Leche League Breastfeeding Hotline: (800) 525-3243
Medicare Hotline: (800) MEDICARE
Medicare/Medicaid Fraud Hotline: (800) 447-8477
National AIDS Hotline: (800) 342-AIDS
National Alcohol and Drug Treatment Line:
     (800) 662-4357
National Alliance for the Mentally Ill Helpline:
     (800) 950-6264
National Cancer Institute's Cancer Information Service:
     (800) 4-CANCER
National Center for Complementary and Alternative
     Medicine: (888) 644-6226
National Clearinghouse for Alcohol and Drug Information:
     (800) 729-6686

National Council on Alcoholism and Drug Dependence
Hopeline: (800) 622-2255
National Domestic Violence Hotline: (800) 799-7233
National Health Information Center: (800) 336-4797
National Heart, Lung, and Blood Institute Information
Line: (800) 575-9355
National HIV/AIDS Treatment Information Service:
(800) 448-0440
National Information Center for Children and Youth with
Disabilities: (800) 695-0285
National Institute of Mental Health Information Line:
(800) 64-PANIC
National Institutes of Health Patient Recruitment and
Referral Line: (800) 411-1222
National Lead Information Center: (800) 532–3394
National Marrow Donor Program: (800) 654-1247
National Maternal and Child Health Clearinghouse:
(888) 434-4624
National Prevention Clearinghouse: (800) 458-5231
National Women's Health Information Center:
(800) 994-WOMAN
National Youth Crisis Hotline: (800) 448–4663
Osteoporosis National Resource Center: (800) 624-2663
Project Inform AIDS Treatment Options Hotline:
(800) 822-7422
Social Security Hotline: (800) 772-1213
Y-ME National Organization for Breast Cancer
Information Support Program: (800) 221–2141

Appendix C: State Health and Insurance Departments

NOTE: Toll-free telephone numbers in listings may work only within the state. Before sending correspondence, confirm addresses and fax numbers.

ALABAMA

DEPARTMENT OF PUBLIC HEALTH
RSA Tower
PO Box 303017
Montgomery, AL 36130-3017
(334) 206-5300
Fax: (334) 205-5609
www.alapubhealth.org

DEPARTMENT OF INSURANCE
201 Monroe Street, Suite 1700
Montgomery, AL 36104
(334) 269-3550
Fax: (334) 241-4192
www.aladoi.org

ALASKA

DEPARTMENT OF HEALTH & SOCIAL SERVICES
PO Box 110601
Juneau, AK 99811
(907) 465-3030
Fax: (907) 465-3068
www.hss.state.ak.us

DIVISION OF INSURANCE
3601 C Street, Suite 1324
Anchorage, AK 99503-5948
(907) 269-7900
Fax: (907) 269-7910
www.dced.state.ak.us/insurance

ARIZONA

DEPARTMENT OF HEALTH SERVICES
1704 W. Adams
Phoenix, AZ 85007
(602) 542-1024
Fax: (602) 542-1062
www.hs.state.az.us

DEPARTMENT OF INSURANCE
2910 North 44th Street, Suite 210
Phoenix, AZ 85018-7256
(602) 912-8444
Consumer Services: (800) 325-2548
Fax: (602) 912-8452
www.state.az.us/id

ARKANSAS

DEPARTMENT OF HEALTH
4815 W. Markham
Little Rock, AR 72202
(501) 661-2000
health.state.ar.us

DEPARTMENT OF INSURANCE
1200 West 3rd Street
Little Rock, AR 72201-1904
(501) 371-2600
(800) 852-5494
Fax: (501) 371-2749
www.state.ar.us/insurance

CALIFORNIA

DEPARTMENT OF HEALTH SERVICES
714 P Street
Sacramento, CA 95814
(916) 445-4171
www.dhs.cahwnet.gov

HEALTH PLAN DIVISION
Department of Corporations
320 W. 4th Street, Suite 750
Los Angeles, CA 90013
(800) 400-0815
www.ca.corp.gov/hpd/health.htm

DEPARTMENT OF INSURANCE
300 S. Spring Street
Los Angeles, CA 90013
(213) 897-8921
Consumer Hotline: (800) 927-HELP
Fax: (213) 897-6041
www.insurance.ca.gov

COLORADO

DEPARTMENT OF PUBLIC HEALTH AND ENVIRONMENT
4300 Cherry Creek Drive South
Denver, CO 80246-1530
(303) 692-2000
(800) 886-7689
Fax: (303) 753-6809
www.cdphe.state.co.us

DIVISION OF INSURANCE
1560 Broadway, Suite 850
Denver, CO 80202
(303) 894-7499
(800) 930-3745
Fax: (303) 894-7455
www.dora.state.co.us/insurance

CONNECTICUT

DEPARTMENT OF PUBLIC HEALTH
410 Capitol Avenue, MS #13COM
PO Box 340308
Hartford, CT 06134-0308
(860) 509-8000
www.state.ct.us/dph

DEPARTMENT OF INSURANCE
PO Box 816
Hartford, CT 06142-0816
(860) 297-3900
(800) 203-3447
Fax: (860) 297-3872
www.state.ct.us/cid

DELAWARE

DEPARTMENT OF HEALTH AND SOCIAL SERVICES
1901 N. Du Pont Highway, Main Building
New Castle, DE 19720
(302) 577-3000
Delaware Helpline: (800) 464-4357
www.state.de.us/dhss

DEPARTMENT OF INSURANCE
Rodney Building
841 Silver Lake Boulevard
Dover, DE 19904
(302) 739-4251
(800) 282-8611
Fax: (302) 739-6278
www.state.de.us/inscom

DISTRICT OF COLUMBIA

DEPARTMENT OF HEALTH
825 N. Capitol Street NE
Washington, DC 20002
(202) 442-9191
www.dchealth.com

DEPARTMENT OF INSURANCE AND SECURITY
REGULATIONS
810 First Street NE, Suite 701
Washington, DC 20002
(202) 727-8000
Fax: (202) 535-1196
www.ci.washington.dc.us/agencylist_28.html

FLORIDA

DEPARTMENT OF HEALTH
2020 Capital Circle SE, Bin #AOO
Tallahassee, FL 32399-1700
(850) 487-2945
Fax: (850) 922-9453
www.doh.state.fl.us

DEPARTMENT OF INSURANCE
200 East Gaines Street
Tallahassee, FL 32399
(850) 922-3131
(800) 342-2762
Fax: (850) 488-2349
www.doi.state.fl.us

GEORGIA

DIVISION OF PUBLIC HEALTH
Two Peachtree Street NW, Suite 15-470
Atlanta, GA 30303-3142
(404) 657-2700
Fax: (404) 657-2715
www.ph.dhr.state.ga.us

DEPARTMENT OF INSURANCE
2 Martin Luther King, Jr. Drive
Floyd Memorial Building, 704 West Tower
Atlanta, GA 30334
(404) 656-2056
Fax: (404) 657-8542
www.gainsurance.org

HAWAII

DEPARTMENT OF HEALTH
1250 Punchbowl Street
Honolulu, HI 96813
(808) 586-4400
Fax: (808) 586-4444
www.state.hi.us/health

INSURANCE DIVISION
Department of Commerce and Consumer Affairs
250 S. King Street, 5th floor
Honolulu, HI 96813
(808) 586-2790
Fax: (808) 586-2806
www.state.hi.us/insurance

IDAHO

DEPARTMENT OF HEALTH AND WELFARE
450 W. State Street, 10th floor
Boise, ID 83720-0036
(208) 334-5500
Fax: (208) 334-6558
www.state.id.us/dhw

DEPARTMENT OF INSURANCE
700 W. State Street, 3rd floor
Boise, ID 83720-0043
(208) 334-4250
Fax: (208) 334-4398
www.doi.state.id.us

ILLINOIS

DEPARTMENT OF PUBLIC HEALTH
535 W. Jefferson Street
Springfield, IL 62761
(217) 782-4977
Fax: (217) 782-3987
www.idph.state.il.us

DEPARTMENT OF INSURANCE
320 W. Washington Street, 4th Floor
Springfield, IL 62767-0001
(217) 782-4515
Fax: (217) 782-5020
www.state.il.us/ins

DEPARTMENT OF INSURANCE — CHICAGO OFFICE
100 W. Randolph Street, Suite 15-100
Chicago, IL 60601
(312) 814-2427
Fax: (312) 814-5435

INDIANA

DEPARTMENT OF HEALTH
2 N. Meridian Street
Indianapolis, IN 46204
(317) 233-1325
www.state.in.us/isdh

DEPARTMENT OF INSURANCE
311 W. Washington Street, Suite 300
Indianapolis, IN 46204-2787
(317) 232-2385
Fax: (317) 232-5251
www.state.in.us/idoi

IOWA

DEPARTMENT OF PUBLIC HEALTH
321 East 12th Street
Lucas State Office Building
Des Moines, IA 50319-0075
(515) 281-5787
Fax: (515) 281-4958
www.idph.state.ia.us

DIVISION OF INSURANCE
330 Maple Street
Des Moines, IA 50319-0065
(515) 281-5705
Fax: (515) 281-3059
www.state.ia.us/ins

Kansas

Department of Health and Environment
Capitol Tower Building
400 SW 8th Street, 2nd Floor
Topeka, KS 66603-3930
(785) 296-1500
Fax: (785) 368-6368
www.kdhe.state.ks.us

Department of Insurance
420 SW 9th Street
Topeka, KS 66612-1678
(785) 296-3071
(800) 432-2484
Fax: (785) 296-2283
www.ksinsurance.org

Kentucky

Cabinet For Health Services
275 E. Main Street
Frankfort, KY 40621
(502) 564-4990
cfc-chs.chr.state.ky.us

Department of Insurance
PO Box 517
215 W. Main Street
Frankfort, KY 40602-0517
(502) 564-6027
(800) 595-6053
Fax: (502) 564-6090
www.doi.state.ky.us

Louisiana

Department of Health and Hospitals
1201 Capitol Access Road, PO Box 629
Baton Rouge, LA 70821-0629
(225) 342-9500
Fax: (225) 342-5568
www.dhh.state.la.us

DEPARTMENT OF INSURANCE
950 North 5th Street
Baton Rouge, LA 70802
(225) 342-5900
Fax: (225) 342-7401
www.ldi.state.la.us

MAINE

DEPARTMENT OF HUMAN SERVICES
221 State Street
Augusta, ME 04333
(207) 287-2736
janus.state.me.us/dhs

BUREAU OF INSURANCE
34 State House Station
Augusta, ME 04333-0034
(207) 624-8475
(800) 300-5000
Fax: (207) 624-8599
www.maineinsurancereg.org

MARYLAND

DEPARTMENT OF HEALTH AND MENTAL HYGIENE
201 W. Preston Street
Baltimore, MD 21201
(410) 767-6860
(877) 463-3464
www.dhmh.state.md.us

INSURANCE ADMINISTRATION
525 St. Paul Place
Baltimore, MD 21202-2272
(410) 468-2000
(800) 492-6116
Fax: (410) 468-2020
www.mia.state.md.us

MASSACHUSETTS

DEPARTMENT OF PUBLIC HEALTH
250 Washington Street
Boston, MA 02108-4619
(617) 624-6000
www.magnet.state.ma.us/dph

DIVISION OF INSURANCE
One South Station, 5th Floor
Boston, MA 02110
(617) 521-7777
Fax: (617) 521-7575
www.magnet.state.ma.us/doi

MICHIGAN

DEPARTMENT OF COMMUNITY HEALTH
Lewis Cass Building, 6th Floor
320 S. Walnut Street
Lansing, MI 48913
(517) 373-3500
(800) 537-5666
Fax: (517) 335-3090
www.mdch.state.mi.us

INSURANCE BUREAU
Department of Commerce
611 W. Ottawa Street, 2nd floor North
Lansing, MI 48933-1020
(517) 373-0220
(877) 999-6442
Fax: (517) 241-3991
www.cis.state.mi.us/ins

MINNESOTA

DEPARTMENT OF HEALTH
PO Box 64882
St. Paul, MN 55164-0882
(651) 215-5800
www.health.state.mn.us

Insurance Division
Department of Commerce
133 E. 7th Street
St. Paul, MN 55101
(651) 296-2488
(800) 657-3602
Fax: (651) 282-2568
www.commerce.state.mn.us

Mississippi

Department of Health
570 E. Woodrow Wilson
Jackson, MS 39216
(601) 576-7400
Fax: (601) 576-7839
www.msdh.state.ms.us

Insurance Department
PO Box 79
Jackson, MS 39205-0079
(601) 359-2453
(800) 562-2957
Fax: (601) 359-2474
www.doi.state.ms.us

Missouri

Department of Health
920-930 Wildwood
PO Box 570
Jefferson City, MO 65102-0570
(573) 751-6001
Fax: (573) 751-6010
www.health.state.mo.us

Department of Insurance
301 West High Street, 6 North
Jefferson City, MO 65102-0690
(573) 751-4126
(800) 726-7390
Fax: (573) 751-1165
www.insurance.state.mo.us

Montana

Department of Public Health & Human Services
PO Box 4210
Helena, MT 59604
(406) 444-5622
Fax: (406) 444-1970
www.dphhs.state.mt.us

Department of Insurance
PO Box 4009
Helena, Montana 59604-4009
(406) 444-2040
Fax: (406) 444-3497
www.state.mt.us/sao

Nebraska

Health & Human Services System
PO Box 95026
Lincoln, NE 68509-5026
(402) 471-3121
Fax: (402) 471-0169
www.hhs.state.ne.us

Department of Insurance
Terminal Building, Suite 400
941 O Street
Lincoln, NE 68508-3639
(402) 471-2201
Fax: (402) 471-4610
www.nol.org/home/ndoi

Nevada

Health Division
505 East King Street, Room 201
Carson City, NV 89701
(775) 684-4200
Fax: (775) 684-4211
www.state.nv.us

GOVERNOR'S OFFICE OF CONSUMER HEALTH
ASSISTANCE—CARSON CITY
410 E. John Street, Suite B
Carson City, NV 89706
(775) 687-3370
Fax: (775) 687-3374
www.state.nv.us/cha

GOVERNOR'S OFFICE OF CONSUMER HEALTH
ASSISTANCE—LAS VEGAS
555 E. Washington Avenue, Suite 5100
Las Vegas, NV 89101
(702) 486-3587
Fax: (702) 486-3586

INSURANCE DIVISION
788 Fairview Drive, Suite 300
Carson City, NV 89701-5453
(775) 687-4270
Fax: (775) 687-3937
doi.state.nv.us

NEW HAMPSHIRE

DEPARTMENT OF HEALTH AND HUMAN SERVICES
129 Pleasant Street
Concord, NH 03301
(603) 271-4688
(800) 852-3345
www.dhhs.state.nh.us

INSURANCE DEPARTMENT
56 Old Suncook Road
Concord, NH 03301-7317
(603) 271-2261
Consumer Line: (800) 852-3416
Fax: (603) 271-1406
www.state.nh.us/insurance

NEW JERSEY

DEPARTMENT OF HEALTH AND
    SENIOR SERVICES
OFFICE OF MANAGED CARE
PO Box 360
Trenton, NJ 08625
(888) 393-1062
www.state.nj.us/health

DEPARTMENT OF BANKING AND INSURANCE
20 W. State Street
Trenton, NJ 08625
(609) 292-5360
Individual Health Plan Line: (800) 838-0935
Fax: (609) 633-2030
www.dobi.state.nj.us

NEW MEXICO

DEPARTMENT OF HEALTH
PO Box 26110
Santa Fe, NM 87502-6110
(505) 827-2613
Fax: (505) 827-2530
www.health.state.nm.us

INSURANCE DIVISION
PO Drawer 1269
Santa Fe, NM 87504-1269
(505) 827-4601
Fax: (505) 476-0326
www.nmprc.state.nm.us

NEW YORK

DEPARTMENT OF HEALTH
Corning Tower
Empire State Plaza
Albany, NY 12237
(518) 474-2121
www.health.state.ny.us

INSURANCE DEPARTMENT
25 Beaver Street
New York, NY 10004-2319
(212) 480-2289
(800) 342-3736
Fax: (212) 480-2310
www.ins.state.ny.us

NORTH CAROLINA

DEPARTMENT OF HEALTH AND HUMAN SERVICES
MSC 122012
325 N. Salisbury Street
Raleigh, NC 27699-2012
(919) 733-4261
(800) 662-7030
(919) 715-3604
www.dhhs.state.nc.us

DEPARTMENT OF INSURANCE
PO Box 26387
Raleigh, NC 27611
(919) 733-3058
Consumer Services: (800) 546-5664
Fax: (919) 733-6495
www.ncdoi.com

NORTH DAKOTA

DEPARTMENT OF HEALTH
600 E. Boulevard Avenue
Bismarck, ND 58505-0200
(701) 328-2372
Fax: (701) 328-4727
www.health.state.nd.us

DEPARTMENT OF INSURANCE
600 E. Boulevard Avenue
Bismarck, ND 58505-0320
(701) 328-2440
Fax: (701) 328-4880
www.state.nd.us/ndins

Ohio

Department of Health
Managed Care Program
PO Box 118
Columbus, OH 43266-0118
(614) 466-3543
www.odh.state.oh.us

Department of Insurance
2100 Stella Court
Columbus, OH 43215-1067
(614) 644-2658
(800) 686-1526
Fax: (614) 644-3744
www.state.oh.us/ins

Oklahoma

Department of Health
1000 Northeast 10th Street
Oklahoma City, OK 73117
(405) 271-5600
www.health.state.ok.us

Insurance Department
PO Box 53408
Oklahoma City, OK 73152
(405) 521-2828
(800) 522-0071
Fax: (405) 521-6635
www.oid.state.ok.us

Oregon

Health Division
800 NE Oregon Street
Portland, OR 97232
(503) 731-4000
www.ohd.hr.state.or.us

INSURANCE DIVISION
DEPARTMENT OF CONSUMER & BUSINESS SERVICES
350 Winter Street NE, Room 440
Salem, OR 97301-3383
(503) 947-7980
Fax: (503) 378-4351
www.cbs.state.or.us/ins

PENNSYLVANIA

DEPARTMENT OF HEALTH
PO Box 90
Health and Welfare Building
Harrisburg, PA 17108
(717) 787-6436
(800) 692-7254
www.health.state.pa.us

INSURANCE DEPARTMENT
1326 Strawberry Square, 13th floor
Harrisburg, PA 17120
(717) 787-2317
(877) 881-6388
Fax: (717) 787-8585
www.insurance.state.pa.us

RHODE ISLAND

DEPARTMENT OF HEALTH
3 Capitol Hill
Providence, RI 02908
(401) 222-2231
www.health.state.ri.us

INSURANCE DIVISION
DEPARTMENT OF BUSINESS REGULATION
233 Richmond Street
Providence, RI 02903-4233
(401) 222-2223
Fax: (401) 222-5475
www.state.ri.us

SOUTH CAROLINA

DEPARTMENT OF HEALTH AND HUMAN SERVICES
1801 Main Street
Columbia, SC 29202-8206
(803) 898-2500
Fax: (803) 898-4515
www.state.sc.us

DEPARTMENT OF INSURANCE
PO Box 100105
Columbia, SC 29202-3105
(803) 737-6180
Fax: (803) 737-6231
www.state.sc.us/doi

SOUTH DAKOTA

DEPARTMENT OF HEALTH
600 E. Capitol
Pierre, SD 57501-2536
(800) 738-2301
Fax: (605) 773-5683
www.state.sd.us/doh

DIVISION OF INSURANCE
DEPARTMENT OF COMMERCE & REGULATION
118 W. Capitol Avenue
Pierre, SD 57501-2000
(605) 773-3563
Fax: (605) 773-5369
www.state.sd.us/insurance

TENNESSEE

DEPARTMENT OF HEALTH
Cordell Hull Building, 3rd floor
425 5th Avenue North
Nashville, TN 37247
(615) 741-3111
Fax: (615) 741-2491
www.state.tn.us/health

DEPARTMENT OF COMMERCE AND INSURANCE
DIVISION OF CONSUMER AFFAIRS
500 James Robertson Parkway, 5th floor
Nashville, TN 37243
(615) 741-4737
(800) 342-8385
Fax: (615) 532-4994
www.state.tn.us/consumer

TEXAS

DEPARTMENT OF HEALTH
1100 West 49th Street
Austin, TX 78756-3199
(512) 458-7111
(800) 252-8154
Fax: (512) 719-0237
www.tdh.state.tx.us

DEPARTMENT OF INSURANCE
333 Guadalupe Street
Austin, TX 78714
(512) 463-6515
(800) 252-3439
Fax: (512) 475-1771
www.tdi.state.tx.us

UTAH

DEPARTMENT OF HEALTH
PO Box 1010
Salt Lake City, UT 84114-1010
(801) 538-6101
www.health.state.ut.us

DEPARTMENT OF INSURANCE
3110 State Office Building
Salt Lake City, UT 84114-6901
(801) 538-3800
Fax: (801) 538-3829
www.insurance.state.ut.us

VERMONT

DEPARTMENT OF HEALTH
108 Cherry Street
PO Box 70
Burlington, VT 05402-0070
(802) 863-7280
(800) 464-4343
Fax: (802) 863-7475
www.state.vt.us/health

DIVISION OF INSURANCE
DEPARTMENT OF BANKING, INSURANCE AND SECURITIES
89 Main Street, Drawer 20
Montpelier, VT 05620-3101
(802) 828-3301
(800) 631-7788
Fax: (802) 828-3306
www.cit.state.vt.us/bis

VIRGINIA

DEPARTMENT OF HEALTH
Main Street Station
1500 East Main Street
Richmond, VA 23219
(804) 786-3561
www.vdh.state.va.us

BUREAU OF INSURANCE
STATE CORPORATION COMMISSION
PO Box 1157
Richmond, VA 23218
(804) 371-9694
(800) 552-7945
Fax: (804) 371-9873
www.state.va.us/scc

WASHINGTON

DEPARTMENT OF HEALTH
1112 SE Quince Street
PO Box 47890
Olympia, WA 98504-7890
(360) 236-4501
Consumer Assistance: (800) 525-0127
www.doh.wa.gov

INSURANCE DEPARTMENT
Insurance Building
PO Box 40256
Olympia, WA 98504
(360) 407-0430
(800) 562-6900
www.insurance.wa.gov

WEST VIRGINIA

DEPARTMENT OF HEALTH AND
    HUMAN RESOURCES
State Capitol Complex
Building 3, Room 206
Charleston, WV 25305
(304) 558-0684
Fax: (304) 558-1130
www.wvdhhr.org

INSURANCE COMMISSION
1124 Smith Street
PO Box 50540
Charleston, WV 25305-0540
(304) 558-3354
(800) 642-9004
Fax: (304) 558-0412
www.state.wv.us/insurance

WISCONSIN

DEPARTMENT OF HEALTH AND FAMILY SERVICES
1 W. Wilson Street
Madison, WI 53702
(608) 266-1865
Fax: (608) 267-2147
www.dhfs.state.wi.us

OFFICE OF THE COMMISSIONER OF INSURANCE
121 E. Wilson Street
Madison, WI 53702
(608) 266-3585
(800) 236-8517
Fax: (608) 266-9935
badger.state.wi.us/agencies/oci

WYOMING

HEALTH DEPARTMENT
2300 Capitol Avenue
117 Hathaway Building
Cheyenne, WY 82007
(307) 777-7656
Fax: (307) 777-7439
wdhfs.state.wy.us/wdh

DEPARTMENT OF INSURANCE
Herschler Building
122 West 25th Street, Suite 3E
Cheyenne, WY 82002
(307) 777-7401
(800) 438-5768
Fax: (307) 777-5895
www.state.wy.us/~insurance

Appendix D:
Federal Offices for Questions
about Self-Funded Health Plans

U.S. DEPARTMENT OF LABOR
PENSION AND WELFARE BENEFITS ADMINISTRATION (PWBA)

WASHINGTON, DC NATIONAL OFFICE
200 Constitution Avenue NW
Washington, DC 20210
(202) 219-8521 or (202) 219-8776
Health Care Task Force: (202) 219-7006
Brochure Hotline: (800) 998-7542
www.dol.gov/dol/pwba

PWBA REGIONAL OFFICES:

ATLANTA REGIONAL OFFICE
(Jurisdiction: Tennessee, North Carolina, South Carolina, Georgia, Alabama, Puerto Rico, Mississippi, Florida)
61 Forsyth Street SW, Suite 7B54
Atlanta, GA 30303
(404) 562-2156
Fax: (404) 562-2168

MIAMI DISTRICT OFFICE
8040 Peters Road
Building H, Suite 104
Plantation, FL 33324
(954) 424-4022
Fax: (954) 424-0548

BOSTON REGIONAL OFFICE
(Jurisdiction: Rhode Island, Vermont, Maine, New Hampshire, Connecticut, Massachusetts, central and western New York)
JFK Building, Room 575

Boston, MA 02203
(617) 565-9600
Fax: (617) 565-9666

CHICAGO REGIONAL OFFICE
(Jurisdiction: northern Illinois, northern Indiana, Wisconsin)
200 West Adams Street, Suite 1600
Chicago, IL 60606
(312) 353-0900
Fax: (312) 353-1023

CINCINNATI REGIONAL OFFICE
(Jurisdiction: Michigan, Kentucky, Ohio, southern Indiana)
1885 Dixie Highway, Suite 210
Ft. Wright, KY 41011-2664
(606) 578-4680
Fax: (606) 578-4688

DETROIT DISTRICT OFFICE
211 W. Fort Street, Suite 1310
Detroit, MI 48226-3211
(313) 226-7450
Fax: (313) 226-4257

DALLAS REGIONAL OFFICE
(Jurisdiction: Arkansas, Louisiana, New Mexico, Oklahoma, Texas)
525 Griffin Street, Room 707
Dallas, TX 75202-5025
(214) 767-6831
Fax: (214) 767-1055

KANSAS CITY REGIONAL OFFICE
(Jurisdiction: Colorado, southern Illinois, Iowa, Kansas, Minnesota, Missouri, Montana, Nebraska, North Dakota, South Dakota, Wyoming)
1100 Main, Suite 1200
Kansas City, MO 64105-2112
(816) 426-5131
Fax: (816) 426-5511

ST. LOUIS DISTRICT OFFICE
815 Olive Street, Room 338
St. Louis, MO 63101-1559
(314) 539-2693
Fax: (314) 539-2697

PHILADELPHIA REGIONAL OFFICE
(Jurisdiction: Delaware, Washington, D.C., Maryland, southern New Jersey, Pennsylvania, Virginia, West Virginia)
Curtis Center
170 S. Independence Mall West, Suite 870 West
Philadelphia, PA 19106
(215) 861-5300
Fax: (215) 861-5347

WASHINGTON DISTRICT OFFICE
1730 K Street NW, Suite 556
Washington, DC 20006
(202) 254-7013
Fax: (202) 254-3378

LOS ANGELES REGIONAL OFFICE
(Jurisdiction: American Samoa, Arizona, Guam, Hawaii, Southern California, Wake Island)
790 E. Colorado Boulevard, Suite 514
Pasadena, CA 91101
(626) 583-7862
Fax: (626) 583-7845

NEW YORK REGIONAL OFFICE
(Jurisdiction: eastern New York, northern New Jersey)
U.S. Customhouse
6 World Trade Center, Room 625
New York, NY 10048
(212) 637-0600
Fax: (212) 637-0512

SAN FRANCISCO REGIONAL OFFICE
(Jurisdiction: Alaska, northern California, Idaho, Nevada, Oregon, Utah, Washington)
71 Stevenson Street, Suite 915
PO Box 190250
San Francisco, CA 94119-0250
(415) 975-4600
Fax: (415) 975-4588

SEATTLE DISTRICT OFFICE
1111 Third Avenue, Suite 860
Seattle, WA 98101-3212
(206) 553-4244
Fax: (206) 553-0913

Glossary of
Health Care Terms

WE COULD NEVER LIST ALL OF THE MEDICAL AND insurance terms out there, but here are the ones you're most likely to run across. By the way, we believe that health care professionals should speak to you in a clear and straightforward way. They should not use jargon. You are the consumer, and health care organizations should communicate in your language.

Ambulatory Care. Services provided on an outpatient basis, as opposed to hospital care where a patient has a bed.

Angioplasty. A type of heart surgery, angioplasty uses a balloon catheter to treat stenosis, the blockage by plaque of the inside surface of blood vessels. States including Pennsylvania, New Jersey, and New York publicly release information about which hospitals and doctors have the best (and worst) track records in Angioplasty and Coronary Artery Bypass Graft Surgery (see below). If you're facing heart surgery, learn about the performance of your prospective doctor and hospital.

Cafeteria Plan. Also known as flexible-spending accounts, these plans allow you to pay for a wide range of medical expenses with pretax dollars. Cafeteria plans are usually set up by large companies for the benefit of their employees. All funds in a cafeteria plan must be spent by the end of each calendar year, or the money disappears.

Capitation. When an HMO or a doctor's group gets a specific amount of money each month to provide care to you, whether your care actually winds up costing more or less than the amount. It's the basis of many "managed care" systems.

Clinical Trial. A planned scientific effort to study the effects of a drug, procedure, or device on selected patients, usually to determine safety and effectiveness.

COBRA (Consolidated Omnibus Budget Reconciliation Act). If you're leaving a job where you had health coverage at a business with more than 20 employees, you are entitled to an additional 18 months of coverage under COBRA. You will pay 102% of the full premium.

Co-Insurance. In a Fee-for-Service plan, this is the amount you pay after you have met your deductible. For example, if the insurance company pays 80% of the claim, the 20% you pay is your co-insurance.

Co-Payment. The fee you pay for a medical visit or prescription under managed care; for instance, a $10 co-payment for a doctor's visit.

Coronary Artery Bypass Graft Surgery. Abbreviated CABG and often pronounced "cabbage." This type of heart surgery reroutes blood going to the heart using vessels taken from another part of the body, to replace coronary arteries that have become clogged. States including Pennsylvania, New Jersey, and New York publicly release information about which hospitals and doctors have the best (and worst) track records in CABG and Angioplasty (see above). If you're facing heart surgery, learn about the performance of your prospective doctor and hospital.

Deductible. The amount of money you have to pay out-of-pocket in a year before a health insurance plan (especially a Fee-for-Service plan) starts to cover the costs of your medical care. For example, you might have to pay $500 out of pocket before your health insurance kicks in, after which the plan pays 80% of covered expenses while you pay 20%.

Diagnosis-Related Groups (DRGs). This system of preset fees is the way the government reimburses hospital expenses under Medicare and other government health programs.

ERISA (Employee Retirement Income Security Act). Enacted by the U.S. Congress in 1974, this act helped to create the modern era of managed care. ERISA exempts HMOs from legal liability for certain types of claims in employer-provided plans. This exemption has become a major source of contention for consumer advocates and legislators. ERISA also gives consumers rights, including a meaningful right of review when benefits are denied.

Exclusions. These are specific conditions or circumstances for which your health plan will not pay the cost of treatment. Some plans make it difficult for you to find out what they consider exclusions.

Exclusive Provider Organization (EPO). This is like an HMO, but it offers a larger network of providers and usually costs more.

Fee-for-Service. Also known as a traditional indemnity insurance plan. In this type of health plan, you can go to any doctor, specialist, or hospital you want. After you have reached the limit of the deductible, the insurance company pays most of the bill, and you pay the rest. (For instance, after you spend $500 out of your pocket to reach the deductible, the insurance company pays 80% of costs, and you pay the other 20%.) Fee-for-service plans have become much less common in the last decade. Today, the vast majority of employees get coverage through managed-care plans.

Formulary. A list of prescription drugs covered by your health plan. If you take a drug that is not on the formulary, your health plan will probably not pay for it. You can call the plan to ask about the formulary; under some states' laws, the plan must tell you which drugs it covers.

Gatekeeper. In a managed-care plan, this is usually your doctor, called your primary care physician (PCP). She watches over your treatment, encourages preventive care, and refers you to specialists and other services as needed. The theory is that you will get more focused health care with greater prevention at less cost to everyone. Some patients, however, feel like they get stuck at the gates.

Health Maintenance Organization (HMO). An HMO is a prepaid health plan. You pay a monthly premium and the plan covers your medical care—from doctor's visits to lab tests, emergency visits, hospital stays, and so forth, as long as you use the medical services designated by the HMO.

Health Plan Employer Data and Information Set (HEDIS). Under this name, the National Committee for Quality Assurance (NCQA) gathers data on the managed-care companies that it accredits. Most of the statistics measure preventive care, such as rates of mammogram screenings and immunizations. NCQA sells the data to many large companies, which compare the statistics for different plans while weighing which ones to offer their employees. The scope of HEDIS data, though limited, is expanding as time goes on.

HIPAA (Health Insurance Portability and Accountability Act). A federal law that protects people with pre-existing conditions who stop working or change jobs. If you exhaust your COBRA coverage, or if you were ineligible for COBRA because you worked for a company with fewer than 20 employees, you become eligible for HIPAA. Under HIPAA, you cannot be denied group coverage because of pre-existing conditions—but monthly premiums can be very high.

Indemnity Insurance Plan. Another name for a Fee-for-Service plan, this traditional type of health insurance is becoming increasingly rare.

Independent Practice Association (IPA). A group of doctors who contract with managed-care plans. An IPA-model HMO often uses "capitation," giving doctors an incentive to deny you care. This differs from a Staff Model HMO, where doctors work directly for the managed care company and theoretically have less incentive to deny care. *See also Capitation.*

Living Will. A document that outlines what medical decisions you want made if you are incapacitated and unable to express your wishes (if you fell into a coma, for instance).

Managed Care. A health plan that manages cost, use, and quality of health care. HMOs and POS plans are considered managed care, and PPOs are often included in this category because they function somewhere between HMOs and traditional Fee-for-Service health insurance.

Maximum Out-of-Pocket. This is the most money you will have to pay in any one year for medical care, including deductibles and co-insurance. The amount is referred to as the "stop-loss point." After you reach this point, your health plan pays 100% of the UCR expenses. *See also Usual, Customary, and Reasonable (UCR).*

Medicaid. The government program of health care for people with low incomes, administered by the state governments under the oversight of the federal government. Benefits and eligibility vary from state to state.

Medicare. The federal government program of health care for those ages 65 and older, and for people with certain disabilities.

Medicare HMO. In many areas, people on Medicare can join HMOs, which often promise greater services while eliminating out-of-pocket costs for items such as prescriptions. In return, HMOs limit the choice of providers. Some HMOs have recently abandoned the Medicare market in regions where they were losing money.

Medicare Part A. Covers hospitalization for people on Medicare.

Medicare Part B. Covers doctor visits and tests for people on Medicare.

Medigap. A plan that supplements traditional Medicare coverage by filling in the gaps to help pay expenses. There are 10 standard policies, called Plans A through J, which are offered by a range of companies.

Open Enrollment Period. The time of year when you may join, or change, health plans. Open Enrollment Periods can take place at any time, but most often occur in the autumn.

POS (Point of Service). A health plan that is similar to an HMO, but with an option for people to go outside the managed-care network. If you stay within the managed-care system, almost all of your charges are paid. But you can choose to go outside the system, to other doctors or hospitals, if you're willing to pay more of the total charges.

PPO (Preferred Provider Organization). This is a modified type of Fee-for-Service plan. You go to a doctor in a network, who is a "preferred provider," and pay a percentage of the bill. If you go to a doctor outside the provider network, you pay more. A PPO is sometimes referred to as "managed Fee-for-Service" and is similar to a POS plan, but with more flexibility.

Pre-Existing Condition. An existing, chronic health problem. If you join a new health plan, it probably will not pay for the treatment of any pre-existing conditions for a set period of time.

Premium. The monthly or annual amount you and/or your employer pay for health coverage.

Primary Care Physician (PCP). Your main doctor. Managed-care plans use this piece of jargon, along with the term gatekeeper.

Provider. Any person or place providing medical care, be it a doctor, nurse, clinic, hospital, etc.

PSO (Provider-Sponsored Organization). Some hospitals and doctor groups are trying to compete with insurance and managed-care companies by setting up their own plans, claiming that they will give you better care because they are focused on medicine. They are not necessarily financial wizards, though, and some PSOs have gone under because of bad management.

Purchaser. Whoever is paying for the care. This usually refers to companies that purchase health care coverage for their employees.

Self-Funded Plan. Some large employers set up self-funded health plans, meaning that they pay their employees' health costs directly, taking the insurance "risk" on themselves. These plans are not covered by state laws, and you cannot appeal their decisions to your state Insurance Department. If you have a problem in a self-funded plan, you can contact the U.S. Department of Labor, which oversees the plans under the federal law known as ERISA.

Staff Model. In an HMO, this means that the doctor works directly for the HMO and receives an annual salary. It differs from an IPA (Independent Practice Association), in which doctors contract with many HMOs/health plans and receive fees for their services and may receive "capitated" fees which give them an incentive to deny care.

Third-Party Payer. Anyone else who is paying for your health care services. It can be an insurance company, HMO, PPO, or government agency.

Usual, Customary, and Reasonable (UCR). If you go to a doctor or other medical provider that your plan considers "out-of-network" (particularly under POS and PPO plans), the plan will reimburse you according to its own fee schedule on a "Usual, Customary, and Reasonable" rate. You will have to pay any difference, which can add up to a lot of money. Get as much information as possible about fees before you visit an out-of-network doctor.

Utilization Review (UR). A method for a health plan to determine whether an enrollee is receiving appropriate care. If you are denied a medical service because of a Utilization Review, you can and should appeal the decision immediately.

Index

Medical mistakes, 42, 96, 105, 111–119
Medical necessity, 39, 64–65, 69–72, 137
Medical records, 89, 135–140
Medical Saving Account (MSA), 53, 171
Medical Society, 158
Medicare, 34, 48, 109, 139, 158, 165–169, 174, 207, 237, 239, 240
Medicare HMOs, 34, 166, 239
Medicare Rights Center (MRC), 168
Medicare+Choice, 166
MedicineNet, 175
Mediconsult, 176
Medigap, 166, 169, 240
Medi-Net, 176
Medscape, 176
Mixed Model, 56
Moody's, 63
Muscular Dystrophy Association (MDA), 199
Mutual of Omaha, 53

N

National Academy of Elder Law Attorneys (NAELA), 199
National Academy of Sciences, 111–112
National AIDS Hotline, 207
National Alcohol and Drug Treatment Line, 207
National Alliance for the Mentally Ill (NAMI), 199, 207
National Alliance of Breast Cancer Organizations (NABCO), 200
National Association for Home Care (NAHC), 200
National Association of Insurance Commissioners (NAIC), 167, 200
National Breast Cancer Coalition (NBCC), 157
National Cancer Institute (NCI), 173, 176, 200, 207

National Center for Complementary and Alternative Medicine (NCCAM), 100, 176, 200, 207
National Clearinghouse for Alcohol and Drug Information (NCADI), 176, 201, 207
National Committee for Quality Assurance (NCQA), 47, 201, 238
National Council on Alcoholism and Drug Dependence, 208
National Council on the Aging, 169
National Domestic Violence Hotline, 208
National Down Syndrome Society (NDSS), 202
National Guideline Clearinghouse, 39, 109, 176
National Health Law Program, 169
National Heart, Lung, and Blood Institute Information Line, 208
National HIV/AIDS Treatment Information Service, 208
National Information Center for Children and Youth with Disabilities (NICHCY), 202, 208
National Institute of Mental Health (NIMH), 202, 208
National Institute of Neurological Disorders and Stroke (NINDS), 202
National Institute on Aging (NIA), 202
National Institutes of Health (NIH), 100, 158, 172, 173, 175, 176, 200, 202, 208
National Lead Information Center, 208
National Marfan Foundation, 203
National Marrow Donor Program, 208
National Maternal and Child Health Clearinghouse (NMCHC), 203, 208

Notes

———

Doctor's Name: _____

Doctor's Phone Number:_____

Specialist's Name:_____

Specialist's Phone Number:_____

Health Plan Name:_____

Health Plan Phone Number:_____

Your Plan Member Number:_____

Pharmacy Name:_____

Pharmacy Phone Number:_____

Medication Name:_____

Medication Number:_____

Medication #2 Name:_____

Medication #2 Number:_____

Medication #3 Name:_____

Medication #3 Number:_____

Notes

JULIE LERNER is a survivor of cancer who learned firsthand the need to be an assertive consumer of health care. Diagnosed with non-Hodgkin's lymphoma when she was 26 years old, she fought cancer for four years and survived two bone marrow transplants. She is now in remission. Julie works as a marketing executive in the restaurant industry, and previously worked as a sales representative for radio stations including WNCN in New York City. She earned a Bachelor's Degree in Radio, Television, and Film from Northwestern University and a certificate from the French Culinary Institute. She served on the Board of Directors of Cure For Lymphoma Foundation, and was the poster girl (literally) for a New York Blood Center campaign.

PAUL LERNER, Julie's brother, discovered the power of patient advocacy during his five years working as an AIDS advocate. He received a Bachelor's Degree in English from Columbia University. Paul worked as an Assistant Editor at William Morrow & Company, and then returned to Columbia as the Publications Officer for the Harriman Institute. After receiving a Master's Degree in Communications Management from the Annenberg School for Communication at USC, he conducted award-winning work as Communications Director for AIDS Project Los Angeles and Marketing Director for Los Angeles Shanti. Paul lives in Seattle.

The Lerners' first book was the acclaimed *Lerner Survey of Health Care in New York: Your Consumer Guide to HMOs, Health Insurance Plans, Hospitals, Free and Low-Cost Services, and Your Legal Rights.*

Order Form

Lerner's Consumer Guide to Health Care is available at bookstores.

We encourage you to support your local booksellers.

For direct orders:
> Telephone orders: Call Toll Free: (888) 9-LERNER
> Online orders: www.LernerHealth.com

Postal orders: Mail to
> PO Box 20697, Seattle, WA 98102

_Name:_____

_Address:_____

City: _____ _State:_ _____ _Zip:_ _____

Telephone: (_)_ _____

E-Mail Address: _____

Number of books: _____@ $13.95 each:_ _____

NY and WA residents, add applicable sales tax: _____

Add shipping:_____
($3.95 for the first book and $1 for each additional book)

Total:_____

Payment: ☐ Check

Credit card: ☐ VISA, ☐ MasterCard, ☐ American Express

Card number: _____Exp. date: ____/_____

Name on card: _____